This book is due for return on or before the last date

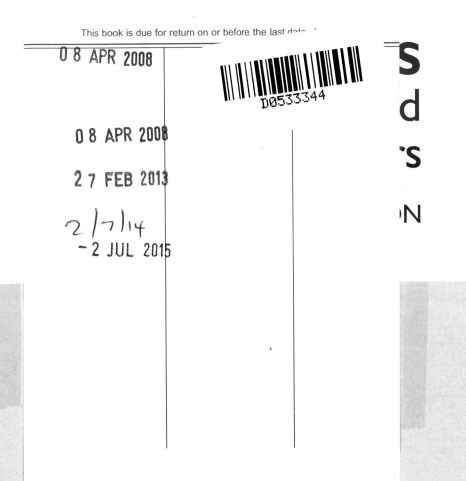

D0533344

S
d
's
N

HOT TOPICS
for MRCGP and
General Practitioners

4TH EDITION

Louise R Newson
Bsc(Hons) MBChB (Hons) MRCP MRCGP
General Practitioner
West Midlands

Rupal Shah
MBBS (Hons) MRCGP DRCOG
General Practitioner
London

Ash M Patel
MBChB MRCGP DRCOG DFFP
General Practitioner
Cheshire

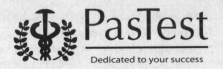

PasTest
Dedicated to your success

© 2006 PASTEST LTD
Egerton Court
Parkgate Estate
Knutsford
Cheshire
WA16 8DX

Telephone: 01565 752000

First Published 2006
ISBN: 1904627 722

A catalogue record for this book is available from the British Library. The information contained within this book was obtained by the author from reliable sources. However, while every effort has been make to ensure its accuracy, no responsibility for loss, damage or injury occasioned to any person acting or refraining from action as a result of information contained herein can be accepted by the publishers or author.

PasTest Revision Books and Intensive Courses
PasTest has been established in the field of postgraduate medical education since 1972, providing revision books and intensive study courses for doctors preparing for their professional examinations.

Books and courses are available for the following specialties:
MRCGP, MRCP Parts 1 and 2, MRCPCH Parts 1 and 2, MRCPsych, MRCS, MRCOG Parts 1 and 2, DRCOG, DCH, FRCA, PLAB Parts 1 and 2.

For further details contact:
PasTest, Freepost, Knutsford, Cheshire WA16 7BR
Tel: 01565 752000 Fax: 01565 650264
www.pastest.co.uk enquiries@pastest.co.uk
Text prepared by Carnegie Publishing, Lancaster
Printed and bound in the UK by The Alden Group Ltd, Oxfordshire

Contents

Foreword

This is an excellent book. I know of no other book that clearly brings together the latest core knowledge of general practice in such an easy to read way. It covers not only the clinical aspects but also the essential wider context in which general practice is organised. It is essential reading for any MRCGP examination candidate but it is also useful for any doctor who wants to know more about the current dilemmas that we all face in our daily work. Reading through the comprehensive chapters is almost effortless but at the end there is a smug feeling of being on top of the subject.

I congratulate Louise, Rupal and Ash in producing another high quality edition. Their hard work certainly makes the work of the reader easier.

John Sandars
General Practitioner and Senior Lecturer in Community Based Education
The University of Leeds
Examiner MRCGP examination

Acknowledgements

We would like to thank our families, especially Paul, Priti and Alistair, for all their patience, support and tolerance over the past months. We would also like to thank John Sandars for all his advice and encouragement in developing this book. Finally, we thank the PasTest Publishing Department, as without their help and guidance we would have never been able to create it.

The chapter on Prostate Cancer is written by Paul CB Anderson BSc (Hons) MBChB (Hons) FRCS (Urol), Specialist Registrar in Urology, West Midlands.

The section on Osteoarthritis is written by AJ Tindall MRCS (Eng.) Specialist Registrar in Orthopaedics, SE Thames.

Introduction

Following the success of the first, second and third editions of the book, we have updated and revised it to produce this edition. We have also added some new chapters on important and topical subjects.

The MRCGP exam seems a long way off at the beginning of the Registrar year, but unfortunately it soon comes round! The amount of information required to work as a general practitioner and to pass the exam can appear to be completely daunting and overwhelming.

When Ash and Louise were preparing for the MRCGP exam in Summer 2000, they were disappointed to find a relative paucity of books and courses to help with 'hot topic' revision. They and other members of their VTS group spent numerous laborious hours trawling through and summarising back issues of the *BMJ* and *Br J Gen Pract*, hoping it would help with their revision, but they found it quite a fruitless exercise. It is also sometimes difficult to prioritise and become familiar with the more important, well-researched papers on a topic.

This book has been designed to help you improve your breadth and depth of knowledge of various important clinical and non-clinical subjects. Medicine is a dynamic specialty and information is constantly being updated and theories altered as more research is performed and attitudes of both doctors and patients change.

It is impossible to predict topics for future exams successfully, and for that reason the subjects covered in this book will be as relevant as possible to present and future general practice. This book is not meant to be a comprehensive revision course for the exam; it is written to provide some guidance and ideas upon which to base your revision. It will also hopefully save you some time by reducing the need for reading and summarising all the journals.

Each of the hot topics is presented as a broad overview with reference to recent literature. References, useful reading material and relevant websites are also included for each topic.

The reviews of various key 'hot topics' are important for both the exam and future careers in general practice. The book is also very useful for established GPs who would like a review of the current literature on a wide variety of topics.

Why bother with Hot Topics?

There are questions in Paper 1 (the written paper) specifically designed to test candidates' knowledge and interpretation of general practice literature. Candidates are expected to be familiar with items in the medical literature that have influenced current thinking in general practice. Paper 2 (the MCQs) has questions based on articles and reviews printed over the last eighteen months. The viva also concentrates on topics that require an awareness of the recent literature.

In addition, good GPs use evidence-based medicine as a starting point and are able to apply it to meet the needs and circumstances of an individual patient, and to reach a joint decision with the patient. A 'patient-centred' approach is a highly desirable quality for the MRCGP exam and for future practice.

Myths about Hot Topics for the exam

You need to know everything

Although the amount of information you are expected to know may feel insurmountable, it is important to remember that it is impossible to know everything, the examiners certainly don't! There is no shame, and indeed much credit, in knowing your own and your professional limitations. Too much pride or arrogance can actually be off-putting to the examiners.

You need to be able to quote papers to pass the exam

Candidates are not expected to be able to quote individual references of articles. It is more important, for example, to know that there are many papers with different results regarding the antibiotic treatment of sore throats rather than to know only one paper and its design faults in detail.

If you know a key paper was printed recently in the BMJ, for example, then it is worth stating. However, it is worse to misquote a reference or quote a reference in the wrong context than to not quote at all! The College states that inaccurate or incomplete references will not be penalised but misleading ones will.

Hot Topics are the most important part of revision for the exam

Recently, more emphasis has been placed on candidates' awareness of current issues for the exam, especially as evidence-based medicine is becoming a very important part of clinical practice.

However, the examiners are actually more interested in ensuring that candidates are broad-minded, patient-centred and can consider problems in general practice from many different perspectives and be able to think about social, ethical, political and cultural factors. It is the application of any knowledge obtained rather than the knowledge itself which is important for both the exam and working in general practice.

Although 3½ hours seems a long time for the written paper, the exam passes quickly with very little spare time. If candidates spend too much time on Hot Topics or current literature in their answers this may be detrimental because it leaves less time to spend on other very relevant issues. For example, when considering an answer about the optimal management of a newly diagnosed diabetic patient, the impact this diagnosis may have on both the patient and their family is equally as important as discussing various trials regarding target glycosylated haemogloblin levels.

Useful reading material for 'Hot Topics' revision

There are a large number of revision books for the exam and a huge number of books about general practice. Your trainer and VTS scheme will be able to advise you about these.

It is generally advised that candidates should be up-to-date with the past 18 months of the literature. However, it is worth bearing in mind that there are many older studies which still influence general practice. The main journals to read are the *British Medical Journal* and the *British Journal of General Practice*, as exam questions are usually set from these and also they are the journals that examiners usually read! *The Drug and Therapeutics Bulletin* is a useful journal as it provides unbiased reviews. The new Clinical Evidence book, produced every six months by the BMJ, is a useful reference source for evidence-based medicine.

The free weekly newspapers – *GP, Pulse* and *Doctor* – contain very useful relevant discussion material, both clinical and non-clinical. Update also produces some very relevant articles and includes self-assessment exercises every month, which consist of MCQs, Modified Essay Questions, Short Answer Questions and Critical Reading Exercise. These can be very useful for discussing with your trainer or in your study groups.

It is preferable to try and read some journals on a regular basis rather than trying to cram everything in the month before the exam. This not only makes last-minute revision less stressful but it also means that some of the knowledge can be used during clinical practice.

Key points

✓ Do not panic!

✓ You do not have to know everything

✓ Try to read journals regularly

✓ Use evidence-based medicine in your practice

Useful Journals/Publications

- ✓ *British Medical Journal (BMJ)*
- ✓ *British Journal of General Practice (Br J Gen Pract)*
- ✓ *GP/Doctor/Pulse*
- ✓ *Update*
- ✓ *Drug and Therapeutics Bulletin (Drug Ther Bull)*

CHAPTER 1:
CARDIOVASCULAR DISEASE

CHAPTER 1: CARDIOVASCULAR DISEASE

The prevention of cardiovascular disease (CVD) is one of the most important tasks for general practice. CVD remains the principal cause of death in the UK – half the population of the UK will be killed or disabled by a myocardial infarction (MI), cerebrovascular accident (CVA) or other cardiovascular event and one-fifth of these deaths occur below retirement age. One-third are considered to be premature – occurring before the age of 75. CVD is also considered to be the leading cause of disability in Europe. It has been estimated that 4.2% of men and 3.2% of women in England and Wales are being treated for coronary heart disease (CHD). The main risk factors are smoking, hypertension, hyperlipidaemia, diabetes mellitus, obesity and social deprivation. These will all be discussed within this chapter.

The medical priority is to focus on those who are at highest risk of CVD. The first priority is secondary prevention for patients with established CVD. The second priority is primary prevention for people at high risk of developing CVD, ie those with an absolute CVD risk >20% (equivalent to CHD risk >15%) over 10 years, as calculated using the Joint British Society's coronary risk-prediction charts.

Hypertension

Hypertension was defined by the World Health Organization in 1993 as the blood pressure above which intervention reduces risk. Hypertension is a very common but poorly managed condition. More than one-quarter of the world's adult population had hypertension in 2000; this is predicted to increase to 29% by 2025 (*Lancet* 2005; **365**: 217–223).

The control of hypertension is still very poor – only about 10% of the hypertensive patients in the UK have adequate control (*Hypertension* 2004; **43**: 10–17). With the increasingly tough treatment targets proposed by the British Hypertension Society (BHS), it is likely that even fewer patients will be 'adequately controlled'.

Hypertension treatment decreases the risk of fatal and non-fatal stroke, cardiac events and death. People at a greater cardiovascular risk when they start treatment, such as elderly patients, derive the most absolute benefit from drug treatment. However, the potential for side-effects such as falls resulting from postural hypotension should not be ignored. The question of whether to start treatment in the elderly should be decided on a case by case basis, taking into account co-morbidities.

By how much should blood pressure (BP) be lowered?

The 2004 BHS guidelines state that:

> ✓ **In non-diabetic patients, the aim is to reduce the BP to below 140/85 mmHg.** The maximum acceptable level (audit standard) is **150/90 mmHg.**

> ✓ **In diabetic patients, patients with established CVD and patients with renal impairment, BP should be reduced to below 130/80 mmHg**. The maximum acceptable level is **140/80 mmHg.**

This differs from the General Medical Services (GMS) contract, which awards quality and outcomes framework (QOF) points for achieving BP targets of <150/90 mmHg (145/85 mmHg for diabetics).

For most patients over the age of 50 years, systolic BP is more important than diastolic BP in terms of risk of CVD.

The BP targets proposed by the BHS are partly based on one large randomised controlled trial, the Hypertension Optimal Treatment (HOT) trial (*Lancet* 1998; **351**: 1755–1762), which looked at outcomes in terms of major CVD events in 18,790 hypertensive patients aged between 50 and 80 who were randomly assigned to a target diastolic BP of ≤90, ≤85 or ≤80 mmHg.

This study showed that the lowest incidence of CVD events occurred at a mean diastolic blood pressure of 82.6 mmHg (and systolic pressure of 138.5 mmHg) and the lowest overall CVD mortality occurred at a diastolic pressure of 86.5 mmHg. An even lower diastolic blood pressure was found to be beneficial in diabetics (≤80 mmHg). Stroke risk was also lowest at a diastolic BP of ≤80 mmHg.

The HOT study is unique in that it was designed to evaluate optimum target BP levels. It also set out to examine the role of aspirin in the primary prevention of CVD, and half the participants were randomised to receive this. Aspirin was found to reduce major CVD events by 15% and non-fatal MI by 36%, although it had no effect on the stroke rate. The benefit of aspirin for primary prevention had been controversial before this study.

What is the best drug regime to treat hypertension?

It is still unclear whether the benefits of specific antihypertensive drugs come from their direct effects on raised BP or from various other indirect actions. However, the overall consensus is that the degree of BP reduction achieved is probably more important than the class of drug used.

Most patients will need at least two medications to control their BP adequately. Giving low-dose antihypertensives in combination is more effective and produces fewer side-effects than a single drug at a high dose (*BMJ* 2003; **326**: 1427).

It is generally accepted that best practice is to choose therapeutic agents likely to do more good than harm, given each patient's social circumstances, preferences, co-existing medical conditions and risk factors. This is also likely to improve compliance. One study showed that only one-third of patients prescribed antihypertensives and lipid-lowering therapy were still taking both medications after six months (*Arch Intern Med* 2005; **165**: 1147–1152).

Some of the most important hypertension studies are highlighted below.

BP Lowering Treatment Trialists' Collaboration
(*Lancet* 2003; **362**: 1527–1535)

Meta-analysis, with data from 29 randomised trials including 162,341 patients.

✓ There were no significant differences in total major cardiovascular events or mortality rates between regimens based on angiotensin converting enzyme inhibitors (ACEIs), Ca channel blockers, diuretics or beta-blockers, although ACEIs reduced BP less.

✓ The conclusion was that treatment with any commonly used regime reduces the risk of total major cardiovascular events, and larger reductions in BP produce larger reductions in risk.

✓ National Institute of Clinical Excellence (NICE) carried out an independent meta-analysis and came to similar conclusions.

ALLHAT (*JAMA* 2002; **288**: 2981–2997)

The ALLHAT (Antihypertensive and Lipid Lowering to Prevent Heart Attack Trial) study was the largest ever hypertension trial, involving 42,000 patients, one-third of whom were Afro-Caribbean. All participants were over 55 with hypertension and one other risk factor. They were randomised to treatment with an ACEI (lisinopril), an alpha-blocker (doxazosin), a Ca channel blocker (amlodipine) or a thiazide (chlorthalidone).

✓ The primary outcome was death or non-fatal MI and there was no difference seen in the three arms of the trial over 10 years of follow-up.

✓ Chlorthalidone was more effective at lowering BP and at preventing CVA and heart failure than the other drugs. There was no evidence of impaired glucose tolerance with its use and it was equally effective in diabetics.

✓ Critics of the trial have complained that it is well known that Afro-Caribbeans do not respond well to ACE inhibition and that this was not taken into account when interpreting the results.

✓ Interestingly, the doxazosin arm of the trial was stopped early, due to an excessive number of deaths from cardiac failure.

ASCOT (Anglo-Scandinavian Cardiac Outcomes Trial); BP lowering arm (*Lancet* 2005; **366**: 895–906)

This large, primary-care-based randomised controlled trial (RCT) involving 19,000 high-risk patients (hypertension and at least three other CVD risk factors) compared two BP-lowering regimes, using either a beta-blocker plus thiazide (atenolol and bendroflumethiazide) or a Ca channel blocker with an ACEI (amlodipine and perindopril). The design was unique in that it looked at combination therapy rather than monotherapy.

The second arm of the trial looked at lipid-lowering for primary prevention in patients at high risk of CVD who had 'normal' cholesterol levels – see Hyperlipidaemia section.

✓ The BP arm of the trial was stopped early after a median follow-up period of 5.4 years because of the apparent benefit of using the ACEI/Ca channel blocker combination.

✓ The BP in the amlodipine/perindopril group was lower by 2.9/1.8 mmHg, which might go some way towards explaining the 14% relative risk reduction in all-cause mortality (number needed to treat, NNT, 125 for 5.4 years).

✓ The primary end point of reduction in non-fatal MI + fatal CHD failed to achieve statistical significance, perhaps because the trial was stopped early.

✓ However, there was a significant reduction in various secondary end points such as total cardiovascular events and procedures (NNT 38).

✓ The risk of fatal and non-fatal CVA was also reduced by 23% (NNT 100).

✓ There was a 32% excess risk of new-onset diabetes with atenolol/bendroflumethiazide. This translates to an extra 4.9 cases of diabetes per 1000 patients treated with the old regime compared to the new one for one year.

✓ Note that only 32% of diabetics and 60% of non-diabetics achieved their target BP (140/90 mmHg for non-diabetics and 130/80 mmHg for diabetics).

There have already been criticisms made of the ASCOT trial (*BMJ* 2005; **331**: 1022–1023). These include the following points:

1. Why was atenolol chosen as the first-line drug in the 'old arm' instead of a thiazide?

2. Why was atenolol routinely increased to 100 mg daily? Side-effects are more common at high doses (including new-onset diabetes) and any increase in BP reduction is likely to be modest.

3. The primary outcome did not achieve statistical significance, albeit because the trial was stopped early.

4. Patients with peripheral vascular disease and microalbuminuria were included whereas patients with biochemical abnormalities were not. This might favour ACEIs over beta-blockers.

5. The differences in secondary outcomes might be almost entirely attributable to the improved BP reduction found with the Ca channel blocker/ACEI combination of drugs.

VALUE (Valsartan Antihypertensive Long-term Use Evaluation) (*Lancet* 2004; **363**: 2022–2031)

This was an RCT comparing valsartan to amlodipine. It included >15,000 patients aged over 50 from 31 countries all of whom had hypertension and were at high risk of CVD.

✓ Amlodipine was more effective at lowering BP than valsartan.

✓ However, after a mean follow-up period of 4.2 years, there was no difference in cardiac disease between the two groups.

✓ There was a lower incidence of new-onset diabetes in the valsartan group (690 cases compared to 845 on amlodipine).

Systematic Review on Efficacy of Atenolol (Lancet 2004; **364**: 1684–1689)

This systematic review examined the effect of atenolol on cardiovascular morbidity and mortality in hypertensive patients.

✓ Four studies were identified comparing atenolol to placebo, including a total of 6825 patients.

✓ There was significant improvement in BP with atenolol compared to placebo, but no effect on all-cause mortality, cardiovascular mortality or MI. There was however a reduced CVA risk (relative risk, RR, 0.85).

✓ Five studies were identified which compared atenolol to other antihypertensive treatments. There was no difference in BP lowering found between the treatment arms, but there was a higher mortality rate in patients treated with atenolol (RR 1.13) and higher rates of CVA and cardiovascular mortality.

This review led to questions about whether beta-blockers should still be used routinely in the treatment of uncomplicated hypertension (although there is no doubt of their benefit in post-MI patients and those who have angina and heart failure). However, there has been some criticism of the methodology of the trial; for example, BP targets were not reached with atenolol alone, and in any case, monotherapy is rarely effective. Therefore, it may be that atenolol was only found to be relatively ineffective because adequate BP reduction was not achieved.

British Hypertension Society (BHS) 2004 guidelines

These guidelines aim to summarise the best currently available evidence on hypertension management. They recommend starting treatment on the basis of risk rather than BP for patients with borderline hypertension.

Important points

✓ All adults should have their BP checked every 5 years, or every year if it's borderline.

✓ All patients should receive advice on lifestyle modification (eg salt reduction and weight loss).

✓ Initiate treatment if systolic BP (SBP) ≥160 mmHg or diastolic BP (DBP) ≥100 mmHg.

✓ Consider treatment in borderline patients (SBP 140–159 mmHg, DBP 90–99 mmHg) if there is target organ damage, diabetes or if their 10-year CVD risk >20%.

✓ Treatment should be initiated according to the 'ABCD' rule.

✓ Aspirin and statins should be considered if the 10-year CVD risk >20%.

✓ Drug treatment is of proven value until the age of 80 years; over this, the decision to initiate treatment should be based on biological age and should take into account the presence of other co-morbidities.

NB.

Ten-year CHD risk is estimated by using the risk chart issued by the Joint British Societies in their recommendations for CHD prevention. CVD risk is equivalent to CHD risk x 4/3.

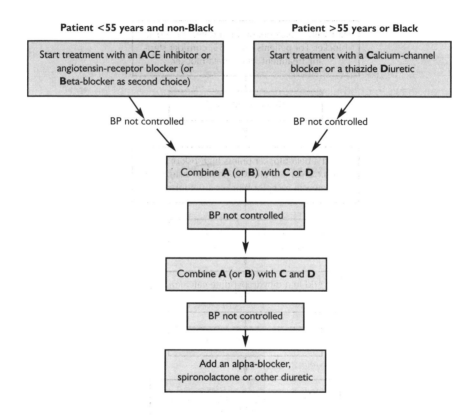

Lifestyle changes recommended by BHS

1. **Salt reduction**. Reducing salt intake to 5 g per day lowers BP by approximately 5/2 mmHg.

2. **Weight reduction**. Each kilogram of body weight lost is likely to lead to a reduction in SBP of 1 mmHg.

3. **Exercise**. Walking briskly for at least 30 minutes most days will reduce SBP by 4–9 mmHg.

4. **Alcohol reduction**. Limiting alcohol intake to ≤21 units for men or to 14 units for women can reduce SBP by 2–4 mmHg.

5. **Dietary modification.** Eating a diet rich in fruit, vegetables and low-fat dairy products with low levels of saturated fat can reduce SBP by 8–14 mmHg.

NICE Hypertension Guidelines 2004

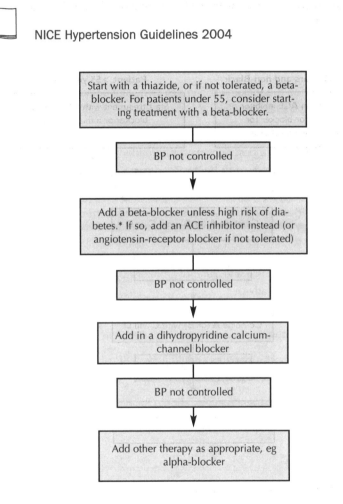

Start with a thiazide, or if not tolerated, a beta-blocker. For patients under 55, consider starting treatment with a beta-blocker.

BP not controlled

Add a beta-blocker unless high risk of diabetes.* If so, add an ACE inhibitor instead (or angiotensin-receptor blocker if not tolerated)

BP not controlled

Add in a dihydropyridine calcium-channel blocker

BP not controlled

Add other therapy as appropriate, eg alpha-blocker

BHS guidance differs from **NICE advice**, which is as follows:

* Do not combine a thiazide diuretic with a beta-blocker in the following patient groups (who may be at higher risk of developing diabetes):

✓ strong family history of diabetes

✓ impaired glucose tolerance

✓ fasting glucose >6.5 mmol/l

✓ clinically obese with body mass index (BMI) >30 kg/m^2

✓ South Asians and Afro-Caribbeans.

It is very likely that NICE and the BHS will issue a joint guideline on BP treatment in the near future, taking into account findings from the ASCOT study.

GMS contract and hypertension

In order to be awarded the maximum number of quality points, practices must achieve the following standards:

✓ There must be a record of the BP of at least 55% of patients over 45 years old within the past five years (the under 45s are not mentioned) in order for the practice to be awarded extra organisational indicator points.

✓ There should be a register in place for patients with established hypertension.

✓ 90% of hypertensive patients should have had their smoking status recorded at least once and 90% of smokers should have been given smoking cessation advice.

✓ 90% of hypertensive patients should have had a BP recorded within the past 9 months.

✓ 70% of hypertensive patients should have a BP of ≤150/90 mmHg (this must be the last recorded reading).

✓ At least 55% of diabetic patients should have a BP of ≤145/85 mmHg (using the last recorded reading).

What should we use to measure blood pressure?

Mercury sphygmomanometers have been commonly used in primary care to measure BP but are associated with bias.

In Sweden and The Netherlands the use of mercury is no longer permitted in hospitals. In the UK the move to ban mercury has not been received with enthusiasm because we do not have an accurate alternative to the mercury sphygmomanometer (*BMJ* 2000; **320**: 815) and aneroid devices can be inaccurate. Electronic BP machines are being introduced in many practices and have anecdotally been associated with higher recorded BP values. One study examined recorded BP in four practices before and after electronic BP machine introduction (*Br J Gen Pract* 2003; **53**: 953–956). No consistent change in mean BP was found.

Home and ambulatory monitoring

Many patients suffer from so-called white-coat hypertension and there is an argument for basing treatment decisions on home readings. However, we should remember that all the major trials that influence our practice today have used BP measurements from the clinic setting.

- ✓ Not recommended in the NICE 2004 guidelines.

- ✓ The BHS gives home monitoring a cautious welcome, but warns against the use of wrist devices. A full list of approved devices can be found on their website.

- ✓ Home and ambulatory BP readings tend to be lower than clinic readings; they should therefore be adjusted downwards by about 10/5 mmHg. Home levels which average no more than 130/85 mmHg can therefore be considered to be normal.

USEFUL WEBSITES

www.bhsoc.org – British Hypertension Society (includes copies of CVD risk charts)

www.bmj.com – *British Medical Journal*

www.bhf.org.uk – British Heart Foundation

ROUTINE INVESTIGATIONS FOR HYPERTENSION

✓ Urine dipstick for blood/protein

✓ Urea and creatinine

✓ Blood glucose

✓ Serum total:HDL cholesterol ratio

✓ 12-lead ECG

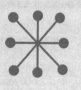

SUMMARY POINTS FOR HYPERTENSION

✓ Hypertension is still underdiagnosed and undertreated

✓ The type of drug is probably less important than the actual BP control

✓ Compliance with antihypertensive medication is poor

✓ NICE guidelines are likely to be reviewed

✓ Many patients need at least two medications

Assessing CVD risk

What are the risk tables – and are they any good?

The risk tables allow doctors to estimate an individual's CVD risk over 10 years, based on their sex, BP, smoking status and total cholesterol:HDL ratio.

The Joint British Society risk charts have recently been revised; diabetes is no longer included as a risk factor, since it is assumed that almost all diabetics will automatically qualify for a statin. There are now only three age ranges: <50; 50–59; and ≥60 years.

Who should be prescribed a statin?

Treatment is recommended for anybody with pre-existing CVD if their total cholesterol ≥3.5 mmol/l. All type 2 diabetics over the age of 50 (or who have had their condition for at least 10 years) with a total cholesterol ≥3.5 mmol/l should also receive a statin. This clearly has huge financial implications.

The new Joint British Societies guidelines recommend that for primary prevention, everyone with a 10-year CVD risk of >20% (CHD risk of 15%) should be treated and that total cholesterol should be reduced to ≤4.0 mmol/l, and LDL to ≤2 mmol/l. These targets are felt by many to be unrealistic.

The NICE guidance on statins for the prevention of cardiovascular events has been produced in January 2006. It states that statin treatment is recommended for **all** adults with a 20% or greater 10-year risk of developing CVD.

Confusingly for us as GPs, other lipid-lowering guidelines do not agree with those proposed by the Joint British Societies. The CHD National Service Framework (NSF) states that statins should be initiated at a CVD risk of 40% (equivalent to a CHD risk of 30%).

At the 30% CVD risk threshold, 11% of the UK population would be eligible for treatment. If the 20% CVD risk threshold were applied, 19.6% of the population would be eligible.

The Joint British Societies charts are based on the Framingham data, which came from a 10-year follow-up of 5000 patients in North America. The risk equations from the Framingham data have been shown to be reasonably accurate when applied to other populations in northern Europe and the USA –

but they have been criticised for not including other cardiovascular risk factors (such as family history, sedentary lifestyle and obesity). They can underestimate risk in:

✓ Ethnic minorities such as South Asians and Afro-Caribbeans who have a high incidence of end-organ damage. A pragmatic approach is to multiply the risk derived from the tables by 1.5 for South Asian patients.

✓ People with a family history of cardiovascular disease.

✓ People with impaired glucose tolerance or the metabolic syndrome.

✓ Obese, sedentary patients.

✓ Patients who come from socially deprived backgrounds; deprivation appears to be an independent risk factor for CHD.

NB.

✓ Patients should still be considered to be smokers for five years after giving up.

✓ Pre-treatment values should be used when assessing patients who are already on antihypertensive treatment. If these are unavailable, bear in mind that the tables will underestimate risk.

✓ The tables can only be used in primary prevention; patients who have already suffered from a cardiovascular event are automatically at high risk, as are patients with familial hyperlipidaemia.

How can risk information be given to patients?

Results of a study from a surgery in London have shown that patient decisions regarding medication are strongly affected by the way information is given to them (*Br J Gen Prac* 2001; **51**: 276–279). A questionnaire was sent to patients asking their likelihood of accepting treatment for a chronic condition on the basis of relative-risk reduction, absolute-risk reduction, numbers needed to treat and personal probability of benefit. The results varied from 44% stating they would accept treatment with a personal probability of benefit model, to 92% stating they would accept treatment using a relative-risk reduction model. In general, absolute-risk reductions should be used rather than relative risk when discussing treatment options with patients.

Hyperlipidaemia

What are the benefits of lowering cholesterol?

In the UK it is estimated that cholesterol levels greater than 5.2 mmol/l are a contributory factor in 46% of CHD deaths. There is now overwhelming evidence that statins are highly beneficial for both primary and secondary prevention of CHD. Target cholesterol levels are achieved in less than 50% of patients receiving treatment.

Certain groups of people are at higher risk of developing CHD and need to be given special consideration. These include:

- ✓ Patients with diabetes mellitus (risk of developing and dying from CHD is two to five times higher than for non-diabetics).

- ✓ Patients of South Asian descent (typically have a 40% greater risk of developing CHD).

- ✓ Patients with familial hypercholesterolaemia (particularly high risk of dying from CHD); the risk tables cannot be used for this group.

Primary prevention trials

There are some key trials supporting the use of statins.

The West of Scotland Coronary Prevention Study (WOSCOPS)
(*N Engl J Med* 1995; **333**: 1301–1307)

Randomised controlled trial involving 6595 men (many of whom were smokers) aged 45–64 years with high cholesterol levels (average 7.0 mmol/l) and no previous history of MI. They received either placebo or pravastatin and were followed-up for 5 years.

Pravastatin was found to reduce the risk of:

- ✓ First heart attack or coronary death by 31%

- ✓ Non-fatal heart attack by 31%

- ✓ Cardiovascular death by 32%

- ✓ Death from any cause by 22%

- ✓ Revascularisation procedures by 37%.

The Air Force/Texas Coronary Atherosclerosis Prevention Study (*JAMA* 1998; **279**: 1615–1622)

Randomised, double-blinded trial involving 5608 men and 997 women with average cholesterol levels of 5.71 mmol/l and no previous history of CVD. They received either placebo or lovastatin and average follow-up was for 5.2 years.

Lovastatin was found to reduce the risk of:

✓ First acute major coronary event by 37%

✓ Incidence of CHD by 40%

✓ Revascularisation procedures by 33%.

Both these studies illustrate that lipid levels alone (except for those with familial disease resulting in extremely high levels) are relatively weak individual predictors of cardiovascular risk.

Secondary prevention trials

The Simvastatin Survival Study (4S) (*Lancet 1994;* **344:** 1383–1389)

This was the first landmark trial of LDL-cholesterol lowering with statins for the secondary prevention of CHD. It was a randomised, controlled, double-blinded trial involving 4444 men and women aged 35–69 years and from 94 centres in Denmark, Finland, Norway and Sweden. Patients were randomised to take placebo or simvastatin. All patients had a history of MI and/or angina and mild to moderately high total cholesterol levels of 5.8–8.0 mmol/l. The patients were followed-up for a mean of 5.4 years.

Simvastatin was found to reduce the risk of:

✓ Death by 30%

✓ Coronary death by 42%

✓ Major coronary events by 34%

✓ Revascularisation procedures by 37%.

Cholesterol and Recurrent Events (CARE) (*N Engl J Med* 1996; **335**: 1001–1009)

Another randomised controlled trial of 4159 men and women aged 21–75 years, all of whom had suffered a heart attack in the previous 2 years and had an average total cholesterol of 5.4 mmol/l. Patients were randomised to receive either pravastatin or placebo and were followed-up for 5 years.

This trial was especially important as it showed the value of cholesterol reduction in patients with what was previously considered to be a 'normal cholesterol'.

Pravastatin was found to reduce the risk of:

✓ CHD death/non-fatal MI by 24%

✓ CHD death by 19%

✓ Fatal MI by 37%

✓ Stroke by 28%

✓ Revascularisation procedures by 26%.

 The Heart Protection Study (*Lancet* 2002; **360**: 7–22)

This is the biggest ever lipid-lowering study and looked at 20,000 patients with a history of ischaemic heart disease (IHD), cerebrovascular accident (CVA), transient ischaemic attack (TIA), peripheral vascular disease (PVD) or diabetes, and included participants with normal and low cholesterol levels.

Participants were randomised to 40 mg simvastatin a day or to placebo for 5 years. Benefits of lipid lowering included:

✓ 12% RRR for total mortality ($p<0.001$).

✓ 18% RRR in coronary mortality ($p=0.0005$). Benefits were seen in all groups, including those with IHD, CVA, diabetics, women, the elderly and those with a low base-line cholesterol (eg total cholesterol <5 mmol/l; LDL<3 mmol/l).

Put another way, 5 years of treatment with a statin prevents a major event in:

✓ 1 in 10 people with previous MI (NNT 10)

✓ 7 in 100 people with diabetes mellitus (NNT 15)

✓ 7 in 100 people with previous CVA (NNT 15).

So convinced was he by these results, that one of the authors made the now famous quote 'statins are the new aspirin'. No benefit was found with anti-oxidant vitamins.

The Anglo-Scandinavian Outcomes Trial Lipid Lowering Arm (ASCOT study) (*Lancet* 2003; **361**: 1149–1158)

This RCT looked at the effect of lipid lowering in high-risk patients with a normal cholesterol:

- ✓ 19,342 patients with hypertension aged between 40 and 79 with at least three other risk factors for cardiovascular disease (but no history of CHD) recruited from primary care settings across Europe (approximately equivalent to a 20% 10-year CVD risk).

- ✓ Of these, 10,305 had a non-fasting total cholesterol level of ≤6.5 mmol/l and were randomised to treatment with atorvastatin 10 mg or placebo.

- ✓ Median follow-up was for 3.3 years.

- ✓ The composite endpoints were non-fatal MI and fatal CHD.

- ✓ There appeared to be a significant benefit from statin treatment; there were 100 events in the treatment group, compared to 154 events in the placebo group (36% RRR for CHD and 27% for CVA).

- ✓ A separate sub-analysis of 2532 participants with type 2 diabetes was also done. Diabetic patients given atorvastatin had significantly fewer total CV events and procedures, such as non-fatal strokes and coronary revascularisation, than did placebo-treated individuals (116 vs 151). This benefit was similar to that seen in patients without diabetes.

CARDS (Collaborative Atorvastatin Diabetes Study) (*Lancet* 2004; **364**: 685–696)

This primary prevention trial involved 2838 type 2 diabetics aged between 40 and 75 with no previous history of cardiovascular disease, but at least one of the following: retinopathy, albuminuria, smoking or hypertension.

- ✓ Randomised to placebo or to atorvastatin 10 mg.

- ✓ All participants had baseline LDL levels of <4.14 mmol/l and fasting triglycerides of <6.78 mmol/l.

✓ Primary endpoint was time to the first occurrence of any of the following: acute CHD events, coronary revascularisation or CVA.

✓ The trial was stopped 2 years earlier than expected because of the benefit observed. Median duration of follow-up was 3.9 years.

✓ 37% rate reduction of a major cardiovascular event over 3.9 years (NNT 31).

✓ This trial supports the policy of prescribing a statin to all type 2 diabetics, regardless of baseline cholesterol.

How low should we go with LDL?

1. PROVE-IT (*N Engl J Med* 2004; **350**: 1495–1504)

✓ 4162 patients with acute MI or unstable angina during the previous 10 days.

✓ Randomised to pravastatin 40 mg or atorvastatin 80 mg daily, for the follow-up period of 24 months.

✓ Significantly fewer people on the higher dose of statin suffered a further major cardiovascular event or died (3.9% absolute risk reduction (ARR), NNT 26).

2. The Treating To New Targets (TNT) Study (*N Engl J Med* 2005; **352**: 1425–1435)

This randomised 10,001 men and women with stable CHD and low serum LDL (mean 2.6 mmol/l) to take 10 mg or 80 mg atorvastatin daily.

✓ Patients were followed-up for an average of 4.9 years.

✓ The mean serum LDL in the high-dose group fell to 2.0 mmol/l, compared with 2.6 mmol/l in the other group.

✓ The high-dose group had a lower rate of serious cardiovascular events.

✓ Interestingly, overall mortality rates between the two groups were not significantly different and the higher dose group may have had a higher rate of non-cardiovascular death.

✓ In addition, there were more treatment-related adverse events at the higher statin dose.

Even when statins are appropriately prescribed, their compliance is questionable. In one study, a quarter of patients were found to be non-compliant with statin treatment (*Pharm J* 2004; **272**: 23). Unsurprisingly, the study showed that the risk of cardiovascular death was higher in the non-compliant patients.

Important additional measures to drug treatment

In primary prevention, smoking cessation alone may often reduce the CHD risk sufficiently to eliminate the need for statin treatment (*Br J Gen Prac* 1999; **49**: 217–218). Other appropriate measures include weight reduction, reducing the intake of saturated fat, regular exercise and, when appropriate, additional measures to reduce BP and control blood glucose.

Diet can decrease levels of both cholesterol and triglycerides. Patients should reduce their saturated fat intake and replace the calories with complex carbohydrates. It has recently been suggested that an 'ape-type' diet, high in oats, almonds, soy protein, soluble fibre and green leafy vegetables, might be as beneficial in terms of lipid lowering as statin therapy (although compliance would almost certainly be poorer!).

Omega–3 fatty acids are known to be important in secondary prevention of CHD, and Omacor (a highly purified and concentrated omega–3 fatty acid capsule, with high concentrations of eicosapentaenoic acid (EPA) and docosahexaenoic acid (DHA)) is now licensed for use post-MI. The GISSI-P trial followed-up 11,000 post-MI patients for 3.5 years and found that Omacor reduced the absolute risk of death, non-fatal MI and stroke by 1.3% (*Lancet* 1999; **354**: 447–455). Omacor is also licensed for treatment of hypertriglyceridaemia in combination with statins and diet.

Which statin should be used?

The *Drug and Therapeutics Bulletin* (DTB) (March 2001) recommends simvastatin as routine first-line treatment; the Heart Protection Study (HPS) would seem to endorse this, as does NICE draft guidance which recommends using the cheapest effective statin. Atorvastatin and simvastatin appear to have the greatest effect in lowering plasma triglyceride concentrations.

Ezetimibe works by inhibiting cholesterol absorption from the small intestine. It is very effective in combination with statins, but is less so on its own.

Patients should be prescribed the lowest licensed dose initially, which should be taken in the evening for maximum effect. Measurement of total or LDL-cholesterol concentrations should be performed 6 weeks after dosage adjustments are made and then annually when the desired lipid concentrations are achieved. Doctors in the UK are very conservative in their prescribing of statins; although in trials simvastatin have been shown to be most effective at 20 mg daily, 42% of prescriptions for simvastatin are for 10 mg daily (*Br J Diabetes Vasc Dis* 2004; (Suppl. 1): S5).

Simvastatin available over the counter

The reclassification of simvastatin 10 mg from a prescription-only medication to one that is available on the recommendation of the pharmacist has raised many important issues about medical practice. The proposal stated that regardless of the pre-treatment level, simvastatin 10 mg daily will reduce LDL-cholesterol by 27% and therefore decrease CHD risk by about one-third. These statements are actually correct (results from the HPS study).

Extending treatment to men at even lower levels of risk will not bring about a dramatic decrease in CHD (at least in middle-age).

One concern about statins being widely available is the ability of pharmacists to assess patients before starting treatment. A particular concern is that family history is proposed as a means of identifying people for simvastatin, whereas in reality this requires medical assessment. Secondly, if a high-risk clinical syndrome cannot be identified, CHD risk must be assessed from the combination of risk factors in an individual – including measurement of BP, enquiry about smoking and age and measurement of both total and LDL-cholesterol. High-risk patients may potentially receive inadequate doses of a statin.

It does not seem logical to take cholesterol-lowering medication without knowing the cholesterol level. Those with pre-treatment cholesterol concentrations above 6 mmol/l (the average level in the UK – *BMJ* 2000; **321**: 1322) need repeat measurements upon treatment as larger doses of statin (and therefore medical referral) are necessary. Self-testing cholesterol kits are both inaccurate and difficult to use.

Simvastatin at a dose of 10 mg is likely to be safe and monitoring of creatinine kinase and liver transaminases may not be worthwhile (*BMJ* 2003; **326**: 1423). It has been suggested that it may be more appropriate for GPs to be able to issue private prescriptions for statins so they can assess risk correctly and then give statins to NHS patients who are below a CHD risk of 15% over 10 years.

One study looked at the cost-effectiveness for the NHS of treatments for the prevention of CHD, including statins (*BMJ* 2003; **327**: 1264). It actually found that treatment with simvastatin was the least cost-effective when compared with aspirin or antihypertensive medication. Aspirin in a patient with a 5% five-year coronary risk costs less than a fifth as much per event prevented (£7900) as simvastatin in a patient with a 30% five-year risk (£40,800).

USEFUL WEBSITES

www.bcs.com – British Cardiac Society

www.pccs.org.uk – Primary Care Cardiovascular Society

www.hyp.ac.uk/bhs – British Hypertension Society
(includes copies of CHD risk charts)

www.bhf.org.uk – British Heart Foundation

SUMMARY POINTS

✓ Statin therapy reduces CHD events

✓ More patients should be taking statins

✓ Target levels are going to be even lower in the future

✓ There should really be no lower threshold for LDL-cholesterol

Antiplatelet treatment

Aspirin

According to the BHS guidelines, this should be prescribed at a dose of 75 mg/day for the following groups of people:

✓ Anyone with hypertension over the age of 50 with a CVD risk of >20% over 10 years.

✓ Anyone over 50 with diabetes.

✓ Anyone over 50 with target organ damage (eg left ventricular hypertrophy (LVH) or renal impairment).

✓ Anyone with established CVD.

The absolute benefit of aspirin in people aged 55–59 years is around two first MIs avoided per 1000 population each year (*BMJ* 2005; **330**: 1442). However, the excess risks of gastrointestinal (GI) bleeding with aspirin are 1–2/1000 a year at age 60 and 7/1000 a year at age 80.

In a recent large, primary-prevention trial among women, aspirin lowered the risk of stroke without actually affecting the risk of MI or death from cardiovascular causes (*N Engl J Med* 2005; **352**: 1293).

A recent *Education and Debate* article has discussed the pros and cons of taking aspirin for primary prevention. In one article, the author believes there should be a public information strategy highlighting the benefits (and risks) of aspirin for older people as he estimates that 90–95% of the population could take low-dose aspirin without problems (*BMJ* 2005; **330**: 1440). However, a second article states that the balance of benefits and risks of aspirin in people aged 70 or over has not been clearly defined in randomised trials, and the benefits do not clearly exceed the risks in younger people without vascular disease (*BMJ* 2005; **330**: 1442).

In a prospective observational study in two large UK general hospitals, aspirin was the causal agent in 18% of all admissions for adverse drug reactions and was implicated in 61% of all associated deaths (*BMJ* 2004; **329**: 15). Patients admitted with adverse drug reactions were significantly more likely to be older and female.

Any dose of aspirin above 100 mg is more likely to cause GI complications than lower doses; according to a recent meta-analysis which included 192,000 patients, the incidence of any bleeding event was 3.7% in patients taking less than 100 mg aspirin and 11.3% in patients taking 100–200 mg. The rate of fatal or life-threatening bleeds was 0.3% in the low-dose group and 0.5% in the high-dose group (*Am J Cardiol* 2005; **95**: 1218–1222).

In a recent paper the authors undertook epidemiological modelling in a hypothetical population of 20,000 men and women followed-up from the ages of 70–74 until death (*BMJ* 2005; **330**: 1306–1308). They found that adverse events such as GI and intracranial haemorrhage offset the benefits offered by aspirin and that it should not be prescribed routinely in people over 70 years.

Dipyridamole

The combination of modified release dipyridamole and aspirin is recommended by NICE for two years after an ischaemic CVA or TIA.

Clopidogrel

✓ According to NICE, clopidogrel can be prescribed for the following patients:

✓ Patients with a history of ischaemic stroke, TIA, MI, or peripheral arterial disease (PAD) who are intolerant of aspirin.

✓ It may also be indicated in combination with low-dose aspirin for up to 12 months following non-ST segment elevation, acute coronary syndrome (ACS) or unstable angina in patients who are considered to be at moderate or high risk of MI or death.

Important papers

CURE (*N Engl J Med* 2001; **345**: 494–502)

This secondary prevention trial looked at combined aspirin and clopidogrel use in patients with unstable angina/ACS. Beneficial for very high-risk patients, but for others the increased risk of GI bleeding may offset the benefits:

✓ 12,562 patients with unstable angina or non-Q-wave MI (ie ACS).

✓ Average treatment period of 9 months.

✓ Composite endpoint of CV death, non-fatal MI or CVA was lower in the patients taking clopidogrel plus aspirin compared to aspirin alone (ARR 2.1% over 9 months, NNT 48).

✓ There were more major bleeds in patients taking both clopidogrel and aspirin.

MATCH (*Lancet* 2004; **364**: 331–337)

This study's aim was to assess whether combination therapy with aspirin and clopidogrel is of greater benefit in preventing vascular events than clopidogrel alone, in high-risk patients.

- ✓ 7599 patients on clopidogrel, with history of recent ischaemic CVA or TIA and at least one additional vascular risk factor.

- ✓ Randomised to aspirin or placebo (to be taken in addition to clopidogrel).

- ✓ Mean follow-up of 18 months.

- ✓ Primary endpoint was composite of ischaemic CVA, MI, vascular death or re-hospitalisation for acute ischaemia.

- ✓ 1% ARR of major cardiovascular events in patients on combination therapy; this was a non-significant benefit statistically.

- ✓ Offset by the increase in life-threatening bleeds.

CLARITY (*N Engl J Med* 2005; **352**: 1179–1189)

This short-term follow-up study of post-MI patients showed that clopidogrel plus aspirin is safe and effective.

- ✓ 3491 post-ST elevation MI patients, all 75 years of age or younger.

- ✓ Randomised to aspirin alone or aspirin plus clopidogrel.

- ✓ Composite endpoints of death or further MI before angiography or occlusion of the infarct related artery at angiography was reduced by 6.7%.

- ✓ Many studies have shown that short-term angiographic findings after MI predict prognosis, so there is likely to be a long-term benefit.

- ✓ Adding clopidogrel did not increase the risk of GI bleeding in this patient group.

Women's Health Study (*N Engl J Med* 2005; **352**: 1293)

This study assessed the use of aspirin for primary prevention of cardiovascular disease specifically in women.

✓ 39,876 healthy women, aged at least 45 years, were randomised to receive aspirin or placebo every other day.

✓ Mean follow-up 10 years.

✓ Non-significant reduction in the incidence of major cardiovascular events in women given aspirin compared with those taking placebo.

✓ This overall reduction in risk was mainly attributable to a significant 24% decrease in the risk of ischaemic stroke.

✓ Overall, the risk of MI and death from cardiovascular causes did not differ between the two groups.

✓ However, subgroup analysis showed that risks of major cardiovascular events, ischaemic stroke and MI were all significantly reduced with the use of aspirin in women aged 65 years and older.

Aspirin versus clopidogrel in patients with a history of GI bleeding

It is worth noting that recent trial evidence suggests that aspirin in combination with a proton pump inhibitor (PPI) may be safer than clopidogrel for this group of patients (*N Engl J Med* 2005; **352**: 238–244).

After 12 months of treatment, the primary outcome (haematemesis, melaena, or a decrease in Hb of at least 2 g/dl accompanied by endoscopic evidence of ulcer or erosion) was seen in 8.6% of patients given clopidogrel, compared to 0.7% of the aspirin plus PPI group.

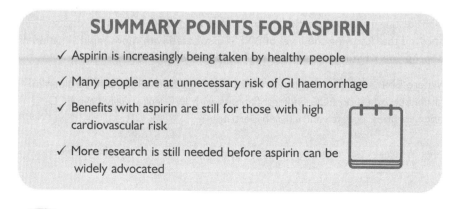

SUMMARY POINTS FOR ASPIRIN

✓ Aspirin is increasingly being taken by healthy people

✓ Many people are at unnecessary risk of GI haemorrhage

✓ Benefits with aspirin are still for those with high cardiovascular risk

✓ More research is still needed before aspirin can be widely advocated

Heart failure

Heart failure, like hypertension, is a very common but poorly managed condition. Fifty per cent of patients with heart failure are undetected, 50% of those detected are not treated and 50% of those treated are not adequately controlled!

Despite improvements in treatment the prognosis for patients with heart failure remains poor: the risk of death annually is 5–10% in patients with mild symptoms and 30–40% in those with advanced disease.

Diagnosis

In their 2003 guidelines, NICE recommends that GPs investigate patients with suspected heart failure by referring them for an electrocardiogram (ECG) and B-type natriuretic peptide (BNP) where available.

NICE suggests that if the patient's ECG and blood levels of BNP are normal, then the patient does not have heart failure.

Patients with abnormal results should be referred for echocardiogram. However, the majority of GPs still have very poor access to out-patient echocardiograms. In addition, BNP testing is still not widely available in the UK, despite being a cost-effective test (*Family Practice* 2003; **20**: 570–574).

BNP is a very sensitive test (90–97%) and if it is negative, then the patient can be reassured that they do not have heart failure. It is not particularly specific however (76–82% specific using a cut-off of 100 pg/ml), so people who test positive do not necessarily have left ventricular dysfunction (LVD), but should be referred for echocardiography to confirm the diagnosis. The new tests have been shown to have negative predictive values of 91% for BNP (*Eur Heart Failure J* 2003; **2**(Suppl 1): 131).

High levels of BNP are associated with a worse prognosis (*Circulation* 1997; **96**: 509–516). A recent randomised controlled trial looked at the larger impact of BNP testing in clinical practice (*N Engl J Med* 2004; **350**: 647). The results showed that knowing the level of BNP is associated with more rapid initiation of appropriate treatment, less need for hospitalisation and lower costs.

Where BNP measurement is not available to GPs referral for echocardiogram should be based on ECG findings. Patients with LVD will usually have ECG abnormalities, eg left ventricular hypertrophy.

BNP value (pg/ml)	Interpretation
<50 in young people or <100 in the elderly	Heart failure excluded
100–600	Borderline
>600	Heart failure very likely

What are the best treatments for heart failure?

There are now so many different drugs known to benefit patients with heart failure that treatment can often become confusing and complex for both the patient and the doctor.

Lifestyle

Patients should be advised to eat a low-salt, low-fat diet, to stop smoking and to reduce alcohol consumption. Alcohol is an important, potentially reversible cause of cardiac failure and one that is frequently overlooked.

It is important to remember that many drugs, including non-steroidal anti-inflammatory drugs (NSAIDs), lithium and prednisolone can exacerbate heart failure. More Primary Care Trusts (PCTs) are funding exercise programmes; a systematic review has found that short-term exercise training has positive effects on physical performance, quality of life, mortality and readmission rates (Br J Gen Prac 2002; **52**: 47).

Diuretics

For many years, loop diuretics have been an important part of the symptomatic treatment of patients with heart failure and fluid retention. However, their long-term effects on mortality rates and other endpoints are not known.

Angiotensin-converting enzyme inhibitors (ACEIs)

ACEIs have been evaluated extensively in large randomised controlled trials. They have consistently been found to reduce mortality and morbidity. Benefits extend to different patient groups: the elderly, women and patients with and without coronary artery disease. Patients with different degrees of functional impairment and with a history of diuretic and digoxin use are also benefited. In the absence of clear contraindications, these drugs should therefore be used as first-line agents in all patients with LVD even if they are asymptomatic.

Despite the evidence for their effectiveness, ACEIs are underused in primary care. Doctors' perceptions of the risks of these drugs in patients with heart failure are often exaggerated; in fact, they are generally very safe (*BMJ* 2000; **321**: 1113–1116). All this is changing with the new GMS contract, in which the prescription of ACEIs for patients with LVD is awarded extra quality points.

Angiotensin-II receptor blockers (ARBs)

It is well established that most patients with LVD should be initiated on an ACEI; and only the 10–20% who develop chronic cough as a result should be changed over to an ARB. However, there is currently debate in cardiology circles as to whether combination treatment with an ACEI **and** an ARB is justified for patients with LVD. For example, recent European Society of Cardiology guidelines suggest that all patients with left ventricular systolic dysfunction should be offered combination therapy with an ACEI, an ARB and a beta-blocker. This is not yet accepted practice in the UK.

The evidence for and against this combination treatment is outlined below.

CHARM studies (*Lancet* 2003; **362**: 759–781)

Designed to assess whether candesartan could reduce morbidity and mortality in three different patient groups, all with symptomatic chronic heart failure (CHF). These three groups were comprised of patients who were intolerant of ACEIs (CHARM-Alternative), patients who were being concurrently treated with ACEIs (CHARM-Added) and patients with a preserved left ventricular ejection fraction (CHARM-Preserved). Candesartan was found to be beneficial in reducing morbidity and mortality but overall mortality was reduced only by 1.6% over more than 3 years of treatment.

- ✓ 7601 patients with symptomatic CHF (New York Heart Association grades II–IV) in 26 countries.

- ✓ Randomised to treatment with candesartan or to placebo and followed-up for at least 2 years.

- ✓ Primary endpoint for each individual branch of the trial was combined cardiovascular death or CHF hospitalisation. Primary endpoint overall was all-cause mortality.

- ✓ The results of CHARM-Alternative showed that after 33.7 months of treatment, the absolute risk reduction (in terms of CHF hospitalisation and cardiovascular death) was 7%; this was for patients who were not already on an ACEI.

✓ Results from the CHARM-Alternative trial showed that people given candesartan had a lower risk of developing diabetes than people given placebo (1.4% absolute risk reduction).

✓ In the CHARM-Added trial, it was found that after 41 months of follow-up, patients receiving candesartan had a 4% absolute risk reduction for the primary endpoint (NNT 25), regardless of the presence or absence of concomitant beta-blocker treatment.

✓ Results from the CHARM-Preserved trial showed a borderline trend towards benefit with candesartan although mortality rates were slightly higher in the candesartan group.

✓ There was an overall absolute reduction in the risk of mortality of 1.6%.

 Val-HeFT (*N Engl J Med* 2001; **345**: 1667–1675)

RCT looking at valsartan use in patients with chronic heart failure. Valsartan found to be of benefit mainly in patients not already on an ACEI.

✓ Designed to evaluate the effects of combining valsartan with standard therapy (including ACEIs, beta-blockers, diuretics or digoxin) for patients with chronic heart failure.

✓ 5010 patients with chronic heart failure.

✓ Mean follow-up of 23 months.

✓ No significant difference in all-cause mortality but evidence of benefit in the combined endpoint of mortality and morbidity (32.1% for placebo group cf 28.8% for valsartan group).

✓ 24% reduction in hospitalisation rate for worsening heart failure in patients on valsartan.

✓ There was a much greater benefit in patients not already taking an ACEI.

✓ Patients already taking both an ACEI and a beta-blocker as standard therapy who were given valsartan had an increased mortality rate.

VALIANT study (*N Engl J Med* 2003; **349**: 1893–1906)

✓ 14,000 patients with LVF following an MI.

✓ Randomised to captopril, to valsartan or to both.

✓ Both treatments were equivalent in terms of efficacy, but there was no benefit in combining them; this resulted in increased adverse effects.

Beta-blockers

Beta-blockers are generally used as second-line treatment, after ACEIs. Only the selective beta-blockers bisoprolol, metoprolol and carvedilol have been used in the large heart failure trials and it is one of these three which will normally be initiated for heart failure. However, if a patient is already on a non-selective beta-blocker prior to their diagnosis, they can continue on it.

Beta-blockers should be introduced very cautiously, starting off with a low dose and titrating upwards over several weeks. An overview of randomised trials found that beta-blockers are generally well tolerated by patients (*Arch Intern Med* 2004; **164**: 1389). It is interesting that in the trials reviewed, more patients were withdrawn from treatment with a placebo than with a beta-blocker!

Recent large randomised controlled trials, CIBIS-II (Cardiac Insufficiency Bisoprolol Trial II), COPERNICUS (Carvedilol Prospective Randomized Cumulative Survival Study) and MERIT-HF (Metoprolol Randomized Intervention Trial in Congestive Heart Failure), have shown that beta-blocker treatment with bisoprolol, carvedilol and metoprolol XL, respectively, reduce mortality in advanced heart failure patients.

COMET (Carvedilol Or Metoprolol European Trial) compared the effects of carvedilol and metoprolol tartrate in patients with moderate-to-severe heart failure (*Lancet* 2003; **362**: 7). It is one of the longest and largest beta-blocker studies conducted in heart failure. The results showed a significant survival benefit of 17% in patients treated with carvedilol compared to metoprolol. COMET also showed that carvedilol was associated with a 67% reduction in risk of deaths due to stroke and a 22% reduction in new-onset diabetes.

Beta-blockers have been evaluated in more than 15,000 patients with mild-to-moderate heart failure in over 20 randomised clinical trials (eg MERIT-HF *Lancet* 1999; **353**: 2001–2007 and CIBIS-II trials *Lancet* 1999; **353**: 9–13). They have been shown to decrease mortality, cumulatively by about 30–40%, and also to reduce morbidity. About 3–4 deaths are prevented during the first year of therapy for every 100 patients treated.

The NICE guideline makes it clear that beta-blockers licensed for heart failure should be initiated regardless of whether or not the patient's symptoms persist after standard treatment with diuretics and ACEIs. Temporary exacerbation of symptoms may occur in 20–30% of patients after starting beta-blockers, necessitating increased diuretic therapy. Most patients in the UK receive either bisoprolol or carvedilol because metoprolol is not licensed to treat heart failure. Like metoprolol, bisoprolol is a selective beta-blocker. No comparison of carvedilol and bisoprolol is as yet available.

The most recent beta-blocker trial is the SENIORS trial, which is outlined below.

SENIORS (*Eur Heart J* 2005; **26**: 215–225)

- ✓ 2128 patients with heart failure (either left ventricular ejection fraction of ≤35% or at least one hospital admission in the preceding year with CHF) whose average age was 76 years at the start of the trial (all patients were over 70).

- ✓ Randomised to nebivolol or to placebo and followed up for an average of 21 months.

- ✓ Primary endpoint was composite of all-cause mortality and cardiovascular hospital admissions.

- ✓ 31.1% of people on nebivolol died or were admitted to hospital compared to 35.3% of patients on placebo.

- ✓ 15.8% of patients on nebivolol died compared to 18.1% of controls.

- ✓ However, starting heart failure treatment with a beta-blocker appears to be as safe and effective as starting treatment with an ACEI, according to the results of the CIBIS (Cardiac Insufficiency Bisoprolol Study) (*Circulation* 2005; **112**: 2426–2435*)*.

GMS contract and LVD

Maximum quality points are awarded to practices who achieve the following standards:

- ✓ Have a register of patients with CHD and LVD.

- ✓ Have echocardiographical confirmation of 90% of their LVD cases diagnosed after April 2003 (in patients with concomitant CHD only).

- ✓ At least 70% of patients with LVD and CHD should be prescribed ACEIs or ARBs.

SUMMARY POINTS FOR HEART FAILURE

✓ Heart failure is underdetected and undertreated

✓ A normal ECG and normal BNP value exclude heart failure

✓ Patients with abnormal ECGs and raised BNP values should have an echo

✓ Many patients are not prescribed beta-blockers

✓ Beta-blockers reduce mortality

Atrial fibrillation

There is an increased incidence of atrial fibrillation (AF) with increasing age; one study suggested a prevalence of 2.4% in patients over the age of 50 years (*Br J Gen Prac* 1997; **47**: 285–289). Atrial fibrillation is an independent risk factor for stroke; its presence increases the risk fivefold. Patients with AF who do sustain a stroke have a higher mortality rate, greater disability, a longer duration of hospital stay and a lower rate of discharge to their own home.

The prevalence of AF increases with age, which obviously means the proportion of strokes attributable to AF also increases with age – about 24% in people aged 80–89 years. However, community-based studies show that AF is still underdiagnosed and undertreated.

NICE has released draft guidance on AF (to be finalised in June 2006). Key points are listed below:

- ✓ An ECG should be performed on all patients in whom a diagnosis of AF is suspected based on the detection of an irregular pulse.

- ✓ The following patients should usually receive rate control rather than rhythm control:

    - people over the age of 65

    - those with a history of CHD

    - those in whom anti-arrhythmic medication is not tolerated or is contraindicated

    - those for whom cardioversion is unsuitable.

- ✓ A rhythm control strategy is preferred in:

    - younger patients

    - patients who are symptomatic

    - patients who have congestive heart failure

    - those who have presented with a lone episode of AF

    - those who have developed AF as a result of a treated/corrected precipitant.

- ✓ There is clearly going to be overlap between these groups, so each patient should be considered individually and the advantages/disadvantages of treatment explained.

- ✓ In patients with permanent AF, who need treatment for rate control:

- beta-blockers or rate-limiting calcium antagonists should be administered as the preferred initial monotherapy

- digoxin should only be considered as monotherapy in sedentary patients.

✓ In patients with persistent AF, appropriate antithrombotic therapy should be administered irrespective of whether they receive rate control or rhythm control.

✓ Patients with AF should be assessed for their risk of thromboembolism (according to the criteria listed below) and given appropriate thromboprophylaxis.

Is rate as important as rhythm?

Traditionally, doctors have concentrated on cardioverting patients in AF, either medically (eg with amiodarone) or surgically, with DC cardioversion. However, drugs that slow heart rate are just as effective as drugs that control rhythm, as well as being cheaper and safer. The key piece of evidence supporting rate control is the landmark AFFIRM study, which was carried out in North America and looked at 4060 patients with AF, followed-up for 3.5 years on average (*N Engl J Med* 2002; **347**: 1825–1833). They were randomised to rate control (with a beta-blocker, a Ca channel blocker or digoxin) or rhythm control. At the end of the study, 356 patients in the rhythm control group had died, compared to 310 in the rate control group. There was no difference in CVA rates between the two groups.

The RACE study randomly assigned 522 patients to aggressive rhythm control or rate control only (*N Engl J Med* 2002; **347**: 1834). It found that rate control was not inferior to rhythm control.

Should patients with atrial fibrillation be prescribed warfarin?

It is recommended that patients who are at high risk of stroke should be identified and targeted for anticoagulation in the absence of contraindications (*Lancet* 1999; **353**: 4–6), see Box on 'Risk of stroke in non-rheumatic atrial fibrillation'. This risk should be reviewed at regular intervals, at least annually. High-risk patients (ie those with an annual CVA risk of 8–12%) should receive warfarin, with the aim of keeping the INR between 2.0 and 3.0; patients at moderate risk (ie annual risk of CVA 4%) should receive either warfarin or aspirin, depending on each individual case; and low-risk patients (risk of CVA 1%) should receive aspirin at a dose of 75–300 mg daily.

Randomised trials have established that anticoagulation with warfarin is associated with a relative reduction in risk of stroke of 68% (*Lancet* 1996; **648**: 633–638). Patients with non-valvular AF who have an INR of 2.0 or greater reduce both their future frequency and severity of ischaemic stroke and also the risk of death from stroke (*N Engl J Med* 2003; **349**: 1019).

Aspirin has been shown to be less effective in stroke reduction among high-risk patients, but is more convenient and theoretically safer then warfarin. There is no evidence that adding aspirin to warfarin confers any additional benefit.

It may be that the thrombin inhibitor ximelagatran will be a realistic alternative to warfarin in patients with AF. Ximelagatran has the huge advantage over warfarin of being a fixed dose and not requiring monitoring or dose titration. The SPORTIF III study was a large study involving over 3400 patients across 23 countries (*Lancet* 2003; **362**: 1691). The results found that ximelagatran was at least as effective as well-controlled warfarin in the prevention of all strokes or systemic embolic events. There were also similar rates of disabling or fatal stroke, TIAs, MI and mortality between the two treatment groups.

Why are some patients with atrial fibrillation not anticoagulated?

Despite evidence in the published literature, anticoagulation is underused in clinical practice. Reasons may include concern over cerebral haemorrhage, the problems associated with initiating therapy in elderly housebound patients and the inconvenience of safely monitoring anticoagulation in the community.

One small study demonstrated that patients on warfarin could manage their INR at home as safely as at a hospital anticoagulation clinic (*Lancet* 2000; **356**: 97–102). This was made possible by reliable, easy-to-use machines using capillary blood samples. Longer-term studies are needed to assess the feasibility of this method, but home management would obviously have many advantages.

One study has highlighted a considerable variability between physicians and patients in their weighing up of the potential outcomes associated with anticoag-ulation for AF (*BMJ* 2001; **323**: 1218–1221). It showed that for anticoagulation treatment to be acceptable, patients required less reduction in risk of stroke and were more tolerant of an increase in the risk of bleeding than physicians.

Interestingly, a recent study has shown that a doctor's experience with bleeding events associated with warfarin can influence their future prescribing of warfarin – those who had a patient with an adverse bleeding event were 21% less likely to prescribe warfarin (*BMJ* 2006; **332**:141).

However, a study of elderly patients in general practice showed that nearly 40% of patients with AF preferred not to receive anticoagulation when they were given information about stroke risk and consequences of treatment (*BMJ* 2000; **320**: 1380–1384). The findings of this study suggest that guidelines for the management of AF should be modified to incorporate patients' preferences in treatment decisions, particularly with regard to the consequences of anticoagulation treatment.

USEFUL WEBSITES

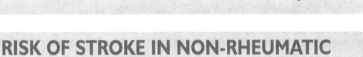

www.bhf.org.uk – British Heart Foundation

RISK OF STROKE IN NON-RHEUMATIC ATRIAL FIBRILLATION

High Risk (8–12% annually)

- ✓ All patients with a previous history of a transient ischaemic attack (TIA) or cardiovascular accident (CVA)

- ✓ All patients aged over 75 years

- ✓ Patients aged over 65 years with a risk factor ie. hypertension, LVF or diabetes

Medium Risk (4% annually)

- ✓ Patients under 65 years with diabetes, hypertension or ischaemic heart disease

- ✓ Patients between 65 years and 75 years with no additional risk factor

Low Risk (1% annually)

- ✓ Patients under 65 years with no risk factors

SUMMARY POINTS FOR ATRIAL FIBRILLATION

✓ Risk of AF increases with age

✓ Associated with fivefold risk of stroke

✓ Rate control as important as rhythm control

✓ Digoxin should be used second-line

✓ Patients at high risk of stroke need warfarin

✓ Ximelagatran appears to be a promising alternative

✓ Patient education regarding risks and benefits of warfarin is important

Coronary heart disease – lifestyle factors

Healthcare professionals tend to overemphasise the benefits of medication (eg statins) and neglect lifestyle factors (eg smoking, diet).

The recent Government White Paper on public health focuses on the following areas of concern: obesity, exercise, smoking, alcohol and sexually transmitted infections (STIs). This White Paper is likely to have significant implications for primary care.

Obesity

Obesity is rapidly becoming a major threat to health. The prevalence of obesity (defined as a body mass index (BMI) >30 kg/m^2) in the UK is increasing; approximately 1 in 5 of the UK population is now obese and this is predicted to rise to 50% of the population by 2030. The prevalence of obesity is already above the critical threshold of 15% set by the WHO for epidemics needing intervention.

Ironically, huge lifestyle changes are rarely needed – 90% of obesity in the USA could be prevented if everybody walked an extra 2000 steps a day and reduced their calorie intake by 110 kcal per day (*BMJ* 2005; **330**: 1339–1340). In other words, 'move a little more, eat a little less'.

What are the problems with obesity?

Obesity results in a huge financial burden to healthcare. Each year 30,000 premature deaths can be linked to obesity; the direct cost of obesity to the NHS is £0.5 bn, while the indirect cost to the UK economy is at least £3.7 bn (*BMJ* 2003; **327**: 1308).

Obesity is a significant aetiological factor in many common diseases. These include diabetes, hypertension, hyperlipidaemia, ischaemic heart disease, stroke, erosive oesophagitis and some cancers (eg breast, colon, oesophagus).

A national birth cohort study found that persistent child to adult obesity is associated with somewhat poorer employment and relationship outcomes in women but interestingly not men (*BMJ* 2005; **330**: 1354).

It is estimated that being obese increases the risk of developing type 2 diabetes by a factor of 12.7 in women and 5.2 in men and triples the risk of developing colon cancer.

It has been recognised for several years that a large waist circumference is also a predictor for type 2 diabetes. Carrying excess fat, particularly deposition of visceral fat, is known to promote insulin resistance and other features of the metabolic syndrome. A large waist circumference is also a predictor for future CHD and should be included in any risk assessment.

A recent case–control study (by the INTERHEART investigators) of more than 27,000 people from diverse ethnic groups across the world has shown conclusively that waist-to-hip ratio is the best measure for assessing CHD risk and BMI is the worst (*Lancet* 2005; **355**: 1640–1649).

Obesity in children

Obesity in children has reached epidemic proportions. The prevalence for obesity is already above the critical threshold of 15% set by the WHO for epidemics needing intervention. More than one in four children in England are overweight or obese, according to a government report published recently which showed that obesity in young people is continuing to rise. Obesity increased most in older children aged 8–10, rising from 11.2% in 1995 to 16.5% in 2003. Levels of obesity were higher among children living in the most deprived areas (16.4%) compared with children from the least deprived areas (11.2%).

Obesity has been found to be associated with certain behaviour in the first three years of life, including watching television for more than four hours a day, having only short periods of sleep and also maternal smoking (*BMJ* 2005; **330**: 1357–1359).

In terms of interventions to counteract this problem, evidence is sparse. A Cochrane review (*2005*, issue 3) concluded that diet and exercise initiatives are largely ineffective in helping children to lose weight and that public health measures may be more beneficial than individual interventions. A school-based education programme to discourage children from drinking carbonated drinks has been shown to reduce the number of overweight or obese children (*BMJ* 2004; **328**: 1327).

What is the role of the primary healthcare team in obesity treatment?

Unfortunately, only one in five obese patients ever receives treatment for their obesity, and those who do have a 90% chance of failure.

Primary healthcare teams often feel very frustrated when dealing with patients with weight problems, mainly because treatment is long-term and relapse is very common. Many GPs feel that tackling obesity falls outside their remit.

A recent qualitative study from London has shown that GPs mostly believe obesity to be the responsibility of the patient, rather than being a medical problem (*Br J Gen Prac* 2005; **55**: 750–754). Many GPs felt that treatment options for obesity are ineffective.

The National Obesity Forum has a comprehensive set of guidelines on the management of obesity in primary care. Points of note include:

- ✓ Involve the whole family.

- ✓ Consider a target weight loss of 0.5 kg per week or 10% of body weight in 3 months rather than using absolute figures.

- ✓ Target other risk factors such as smoking and alcohol.

- ✓ Adapt physical activity to lifestyle.

- ✓ Aim for 30–40 minutes of exercise for 5 days a week.

- ✓ Tailor dietary advice to the individual.

- ✓ Reduce time spent watching television and on other sedentary activities.

- ✓ If lifestyle interventions have not worked after 3–6 months, consider medication or referral.

The Atkins diet

This is mentioned here because of its huge popularity. It advocates high protein and fat intake with low carbohydrates. It allows quick weight loss and certainly appears to be more effective than conventional low-fat diets after six months according to two randomised controlled trials (*N Engl J Med* 2003; **348**: 2074–2081 and *N Engl J Med* 2003; **348**: 2082–2090); however, most of the weight is usually regained within a year. The first of these trials included only 79 patients, and it is difficult to draw any firm conclusions from it in terms of the diet's long-term safety profile; in particular, effects on the kidneys and vitamin deficiencies (fruit is not allowed). In the trials so far, it appears that there is no significant increase in total cholesterol, BP or fasting glucose levels (insulin resistance may even be decreased). HDL levels seem to be improved by the Atkins diet (*Bandolier* review July 2003). Until there is more safety data, it should not be recommended in preference to conventional low-calorie, low-fat diets.

What drugs are available to treat obesity?

There are currently two medications available for managing obesity: orlistat and sibutramine. A systematic review found estimates of weight loss relative to placebo were 4.45 kg for sibutramine and 2.89 kg for orlistat (*Ann Intern Med* 2005; **142**: 532).

Orlistat

Orlistat is an intestinal lipase inhibitor that blocks the absorption of about 30% of dietary fat. In clinical trials of up to two years' duration it resulted in an average weight loss of about 10%, compared with 6% in the placebo group (*Lancet* 1998; **352**: 167–172). Other benefits include a reduction in LDL and total cholesterol, a reduction in BP and improvements in insulin resistance and blood glucose control in diabetic patients.

The licensing criteria for the drug require patients to lose at least 2.5 kg in the 4 weeks prior to starting treatment, and they should only continue with the drug if they achieve a weight loss of at least a further 5% of their body weight after the first 12 weeks of treatment and a cumulative weight loss of at least 10% after the first 6 months.

There may be other advantages of orlistat; the XENDOS study has supported the use of orlistat for obese patients for the prevention of type 2 diabetes in the future (*Diabetes Care* 2004; **27**: 155). Patients who took orlistat for the three-year duration of the study had a greater weight loss. The incidence of diabetes after four years was 6.2% in the treatment group compared to 9% in the placebo group. However, there was a large drop-out rate in this study (66%), which may be due to side-effects of the medication.

Sibutramine

Sibutramine works by inhibiting the reuptake of the neurotransmitters noradrenaline and serotonin, thereby leading to increased feelings of satiety after eating. Treatment with sibutramine has resulted in clinically significant weight loss during short-term therapy (3 months) in obese adults with a range of cardiovascular risk factors (*J Hum Hypertens* 2005; **19**: 737).

The STORM (Sibutramine Trial of Obesity Reduction and Maintenance) trial aimed to test whether treatment with sibutramine could prevent weight regain among patients who had already achieved a weight loss of more than 5% of their body weight (*Lancet* 2000; **356**: 2119–2125). The study showed that 43% of the patients treated with sibutramine maintained at least 80% of their weight loss, compared with only 16% in the placebo group.

In addition, significant changes in cardiovascular disease risk factors were noted, including reduced triglyceride concentrations, increased HDL-cholesterol concentrations and reduced cholesterol:HDL-cholesterol ratio.

A systematic review has shown that sibutramine is effective at reducing and maintaining weight loss when compared with placebo (*Arch Intern Med* 2004; **164**: 994). There is still insufficient evidence to support the long-term risk–benefit profile for sibutramine though.

The UK licence for sibutramine specifies a maximum treatment period of 12 months. NICE advises similar prescribing guidelines as for orlistat (although no initial weight loss is necessary and it can be used in people with a BMI $\geq$27 kg/m^2 if they have a co-morbidity).

Rimonabant is the first in a new class of anti-obesity drug, which targets cannabinoid receptors. In the first clinical trial in obese humans, it induced a modest weight loss and also had a notable and beneficial impact on waist circumference, cholesterol, triglycerides and insulin resistance compared with placebo (*Lancet* 2005; **365**: 1389).

Sedentary lifestyle

Physical inactivity roughly doubles the risk of CHD and is also a major risk factor for stroke. Regular exercise has numerous benefits, including reducing hypertension and CHD and elevating HDL. Short bouts of exercise (for at least 20 minutes) can be just as effective at protecting the heart as longer workouts if done regularly.

The government aims to ensure that 50% of the population achieve adequate levels of physical activity by 2010. However, the second Wanless report (2004) concluded that subsiding gym membership is a poor use of public money.

Diet

Folic acid and B vitamins antagonise the effect of homocysteine. A meta-analysis concluded that there was a significant, positive association between homocysteine levels and cardiovascular disease (*BMJ* 2002; **355**: 12606). Folic acid should be given for patients with elevated homocysteine levels.

There is some evidence that eating a 'Mediterranean diet' reduces mortality (*BMJ* 2005; **330**: 991–994).

Deprivation

Deprivation is known to double the risk of CHD; this is equivalent to the increased risk produced by smoking.

Why are patients not more motivated in reducing their risk of CHD?

One of the biggest barriers for implementing evidence-based practice may be convincing patients that they need to take part in lifelong measures for the prevention of CHD. Patients often perceive a 'heart attack' to be an acute, self-limiting condition rather than the onset of a high-risk chronic disease.

A very interesting qualitative study looked at identifying factors influencing the use of health services by people with angina (BMJ 2001; **323**: 214–217). It found that fear, denial and low expectations in patients from lower socioeconomic classes are important barriers to accessing health services. This may also account for some of the regional and socioeconomic differences in the incidence and prevalence of CHD in the UK.

USEFUL WEBSITES

www.nice.org.uk – NICE guidelines

www.nao.gov.uk – 'Tackling Obesity in England' report

www.nationalobesityforum.org.uk – National Obesity Forum

The report, *Health Survey for England: Obesity Among Children Under 11,* is available at www.dh.gov.uk

House of Commons Health Committee. *Obesity.* London: Stationery Office, 2004. (Third report of session 2003–04.) Publications.parliament.uk/pa/ cm200304/cmselect/cmhealth/23/23.pdf

SUMMARY POINTS FOR OBESITY

✓ Obesity is huge financial burden to healthcare

✓ Variation in management of obesity in primary care

✓ Childhood obesity is dramatically increasing

✓ Anti-obesity drugs have a role

✓ Long-term data on drugs are still lacking

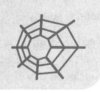

Stroke and TIA

In England and Wales 110,000 new cases of stroke and 30,000 TIAs are estimated to occur every year. Stroke is also the leading cause of disability in the UK, with about 25–30% of stroke survivors remaining permanently disabled and more than 50% being physically dependent on others 6 months after their stroke.

The cost to the NHS and Social Services of stroke is about £2.3b per year; nearly twice that for coronary heart disease. However, the government and charities spend around £5m per year on stroke research, compared to £43m on heart disease. Stroke prevention is actually one of the most cost-effective of all cardiovascular interventions in primary care.

Stroke can occur at any age, but half of all strokes occur in people over 70 years old. With the increasing life expectancy in the UK, it has been estimated that there will be a 30% absolute increase in the number of patients experiencing their first stroke in 2010 compared with 1983.

National clinical guidelines for cerebrovascular accident (CVA) 2004

✓ All patients with acute CVA should be referred to hospital. In the case of a TIA, outpatient review should take place within 7 days.

✓ CVA (with ischaemic aetiology) and TIA patients should receive 300 mg aspirin as soon as possible after their symptoms have stabilised.

✓ A few centres offer thrombolysis for ischaemic CVA; this must be given within six hours of the onset of symptoms.

✓ After the initial dose of 300 mg, aspirin should be continued at a dose of 75 mg per day.

✓ Clopidogrel alone can be used in aspirin-intolerant patients.

✓ Lower BP to ≤140/85 mmHg (or to 130/80 mmHg in diabetic patients). This should only be done in the acute phase if there are likely to be complications from hypertension, eg hypertensive encephalopathy. Otherwise hypertension persisting for more than two weeks should be treated.

✓ All CVA and TIA patients with a cholesterol >3.5 mmol/l should be offered a statin unless contraindicated. This is in order to reduce the risk of a further CVA, but also to reduce the risk of MI; most patients who have had a CVA have a ≥30% 10-year risk of CHD.

✓ Check for atrial fibrillation and, if present, consider warfarin.

✓ Arrange a carotid ultrasound; endarterectomy is more beneficial if done within 12 weeks of a TIA.

✓ Other lifestyle factors are, as usual, very important: smoking, obesity, lack of exercise, salt in the diet (limit to <6 g/day), etc.

Depression is common in stroke patients; it is always a good idea to screen for this.

Prognosis

Patients who have had a stroke have a 30–43% risk of having another stroke within five years. TIA patients have a 20% risk of having a full stroke within the first month. Aggressive control of risk factors is therefore very important, blood pressure being the most important one.

A new risk score has recently been proposed to help GPs decide which TIA patients are likely to be at highest risk of going on to suffer a full stroke within a week (*Lancet* 2005; **366**: 29–36). Patients with a score of 6 were found to have a 31.4% 7-day stroke risk (compared to 12.1% with a score of 5) and should therefore be referred for in-patient care. The scoring system was developed after analysing data from 209 TIA patients enrolled in the Oxford Community Stroke Project. Of the patients who had a CVA in the 7 days following their TIA, none had a score of less than 4.

Scoring table

Factor	Score
A Age > 60	1
B BP > 140 mmHg systolic or > 90 mmHg diastolic	1
C Clinical features	
Unilateral weakness	2
Speech disturbance without weakness	1
Other	0
D Duration of symptoms in minutes	
≥ 60	2
10–59	1
<10	0

What is the value of stroke units?

Stroke unit care is one of the most powerful interventions available to help stroke patients. Hospitals with an acute stroke unit were associated with an 11% lower odds of death in hospital, whereas hospitals that have rehabilitation stroke units or combined acute and rehabilitation units have no significant difference in the odds of death (*BMJ* 2004; **328**: 369). The National Sentinel Audit of Stroke has found that stroke services in the NHS have improved considerably in recent years, but capacity remains inadequate to meet the needs of all patients (*BMJ* 2004; **329**: 426).

The risk of death for patients who received stroke unit care has been estimated to be approximately 75% that of the risk for those having no stroke unit care (*Stroke* 2005; **36**: 103–106).

National Service Framework for elderly people and stroke

Stroke is covered in Standard Five of the NSF. This aims to reduce the incidence of stroke in the population and ensure that those who have had a stroke have prompt access to integrated stroke-care services (ie on a stroke unit). It states there are four key areas for the development of integrated stroke services: namely, prevention, immediate care, early and continuing rehabilitation and long-term support.

Supporting carers

Key evidence includes a trial showing that training carers of stroke patients during the rehabilitation period on issues such as incontinence care improves psychosocial outcomes in carers and in patients (*BMJ* 2004; **328**: 1099–1101).

Another recent study showed that emotional and mental problems tend to be even more pronounced in carers than patients; whereas patients gradually adapt to the new situation, it may become more demanding for caregivers (*Stroke* 2005; **36**: 803–808).

GMS contract and cerebrovascular disease

In order to be awarded maximum quality points, practices must achieve the following standards:

✓ There must be a register of all patients with stroke or TIA.

✓ At least 80% of patients who have had a CVA after April 2003 should have been referred for a CT brain scan to confirm the diagnosis.

✓ 90% of patients should have had their smoking status recorded within the past 15 months (except for people who have never smoked, when a single recording will suffice) and 70% of smokers should have been offered smoking cessation advice.

✓ BP should have been recorded at least once in the past 15 months in 90% of patients.

✓ 70% of patients should have a BP of <150/90 mmHg.

✓ 90% of patients should have had their cholesterol checked in the past 15 months and this should be ≤5 mmol/l in 60% of people.

✓ 90% of patients with non-haemorrhagic CVA should be on aspirin or equivalent.

✓ 85% of patients should have a record of influenza immunisation in the preceding year.

Key evidence

PROGRESS (*Lancet* 2001; **358**: 1026–1027)

This trial clarified the importance of lowering blood pressure in clinically stable patients with a history of cerebrovascular disease. Combination treatment with indapamide plus perindopril was significantly more effective than perindopril alone. There were no data on the efficacy of indapamide alone.

✓ 6105 patients with a history of cerebrovascular disease.

✓ Randomised to treatment with perindopril ±indapamide or to placebo.

✓ Followed-up for an average of 3.9 years.

✓ Primary endpoint was incidence of fatal/non-fatal CVA.

✓ Active treatment reduced BP by 9/4 mmHg.

✓ 13.8% of patients on placebo had a CVA in the follow-up period compared to 10.1% of patients given active treatment.

✓ Separate subgroup analyses revealed that combination treatment reduced BP by 12/5 mmHg.

✓ Only 8.5% of people in the combination group suffered from a CVA (NNT 17), compared to 12.3% of patients taking perindopril only.

✓ Active treatment reduced the relative risk of CVA in hypertensive and normotensive patients by similar amounts. Patients with hypertension had greater absolute risk reductions in CVA risk.

A possible conclusion of the PROGRESS trial is that the benefit seen with active treatment was largely attributable to indapamide; a flaw of the study is that there was no group given indapamide alone. Another flaw is that patients were given single or combination treatment at the discretion of the physician and not randomly; the two groups cannot therefore be directly compared. Also patients were generally younger than the average primary care CVA patient.

HOPE CVA subgroup analysis (*BMJ* 2002; **324**: 699)

The HOPE trial looked at the role of ramipril in prevention of CVD in high-risk patients and diabetics. This subgroup analysis used data from the original HOPE study.

✓ 9297 patients over 55 years with pre-existing vascular disease or diabetes plus another risk factor.

✓ Patients were given either ramipril 10 mg or placebo in addition to their existing treatment.

✓ Only a modest reduction in BP was seen (mean reduction 3.8/2.8 mmHg).

✓ The incidence of fatal and non-fatal CVA was significantly lower in the treatment group than in the placebo group.

✓ Equivalent to an NNT of about 167 for 4.5 years to prevent one stroke.

✓ ACE inhibitors may have some preventative effect over and above their BP-lowering effect, possibly due to anti-inflammatory and anti-oxidant effects on the vessel wall.

Evidence for lipid lowering

In the face of recent results, definitions of hypercholesterolaemia in any patient with stroke or TIA seem artificial. Almost all patients may benefit from treatment to reduce cholesterol.

Meta-analysis of lipid lowering in stroke in patients with or without CHD (*Am J Med* 2004; **117**: 596–606)

✓ 65 RCTs included, with 200,607 patients.

✓ Treatment with a statin decreased the risk of fatal and non-fatal CVA by approximately 25% in patients with or without CHD.

✓ For patients at low risk (<0.2% per year), this equals one less CVA per 2778 patients treated for one year.

✓ For those at high risk (0.9% per year) the benefit was one less CVA for 617 patients treated for one year. Slightly less benefit was found in higher quality studies.

✓ Treatment with diet alone did not affect CVA risk.

See also Heart Protection Study in 'Hyperlipidaemia' section above.

USEFUL WEBSITES

www.rcplondon.ac.uk/pubs/strokeaudit01–02.pbf – Summary report on the National Sentinel Stroke Audit, Royal College of Physicians

www.dcn.ed.ac.uk/csrg/ – Cochrane Stroke group website
www.nottingham.ac.uk/stroke-medicine/ – British Association of Stroke Physicians

www.doh.gov.uk – National Service Framework for Older People

www.stroke.org.uk – The UK Stroke Association

SUMMARY POINTS FOR STROKE

✓ Hypertension must be controlled

✓ Secondary prevention is very important

✓ Lower threshold for prescribing statins

✓ Stroke registers need to be updated regularly

✓ All patients should be managed in stroke units

✓ RCP guidelines should be used

CHAPTER 2: DIABETES MELLITUS

CHAPTER 2: DIABETES MELLITUS

The prevalence of diagnosed diabetes within the UK is about 3%. The incidence is rising, especially as a result of the expanding ageing population and an increasing incidence of obesity. Up to 25% of people of Asian origin >60 years have diabetes.

Diabetes is a leading cause of blindness, kidney failure and limb amputation and greatly increases the risk of coronary heart disease and stroke. It accounts for >8% of the acute sector costs – it has been estimated that the average cost of inpatient care for a diabetic patient is more than six times that for a non-diabetic.

How is the diagnosis of diabetes confirmed?

The WHO criteria for the definition, diagnosis and classification of diabetes are as follows:

With symptoms (polyuria, thirst, unexplained weight loss):

- ✓ A random venous plasma glucose concentration ≥11.1 mmol/l, **or**

- ✓ A fasting venous plasma glucose concentration ≥7.0 mmol/l, **or**

- ✓ A 2-h venous plasma glucose concentration ≥11.1 mmol/l 2 hours after 75-g anhydrous glucose in an oral glucose tolerance test (OGTT).

With no symptoms:

- ✓ Diagnosis must not be based on a single glucose measurement. At least one additional glucose result on another day is essential to confirm the diagnosis. This can be fasting, from a random sample or from the 2-h OGTT. If the fasting or random values are not diagnostic, the 2-h value should be used.

What are the implications of the National Service Framework (NSF) for diabetes?

The Standards for the NSF were published in December 2001 and the delivery strategy in January 2003. Key proposals of the diabetes delivery strategy are as follows:

- ✓ Regular (annual) check-ups for everyone with diabetes to detect complications early.

- ✓ Systematic eye screening programme to national standards (100% coverage by 2007).

- ✓ Local diabetes networks (including diabetic patients) should be set up to plan local services.

- ✓ All diabetics should be on a practice-based register.

- ✓ Systematic treatment regimens.

There is no mention of screening, which was widely expected, especially for high-risk people, such as South Asians. Also, perhaps in response to previous criticism, the NSF leaves it up to Primary Care Trusts (PCTs) to decide on the best approach for local delivery of care.

Diabetes UK has welcomed the NSF, but has raised concerns about the lack of benchmarks (apart from eye screening and regular check-ups).

The routine care of most patients with diabetes is likely to take place in primary care; payment for this is part of the quality framework of the new contract (see below).

What are the Standards of the NSF?

There are 12 Standards presented:

1. Prevention of type 2 diabetes

2. Identification of people with diabetes

3. Empowering people with diabetes

4. Clinical care of adults with diabetes

5. & 6. Clinical care of children and young people

7. Management of diabetic emergencies

8. Care of diabetics during their admission

9. Diabetics and pregnancy

10., 11. & 12. Detection and management of long-term complications.

Since the introduction of the NSF, there has been a major improvement in implementation of structured programmes to support patient self-management:

✓ DAFNE (Dose Adjustment For Normal Eating) for type 1 diabetics (*BMJ* 2002; **325**: 746). This is a course teaching flexible intensive insulin treatment combining dietary freedom and insulin adjustment. It can improve both glycaemic control and quality of life for patients with type 1 diabetes.

✓ DESMOND (Diabetes Education and Self-Management for Ongoing and Newly Diagnosed) for type 2 diabetics. This trial will chart the progress of a group of patients following structured group education programmes and a group who are not. The results of the year-long trial will then be used to compile the first nationally recognised guidelines for managing type 2 diabetes.

National Institute for Clinical Excellence (NICE) has recommended that type 2 diabetics should have eye tests and renal function tests annually. GPs should also be screening all type 2 diabetics for microalbuminuria annually, ideally with an early morning urine test for albumin to creatinine ratio. If this ratio is above 2.5 mg/mmol in men or 3.5 mg/mmol in women on two different occasions, further assessment should take place.

Diabetes and the General Medical Services (GMS) contract

In order to be awarded maximum quality points, practices must achieve the following standards which apply to both type 1 and type 2 diabetics:

✓ There should be a diabetic register in place.

✓ A body mass index (BMI) should have been recorded for 90% of patients within the previous 15 months.

✓ 90% of patients should have had their smoking status recorded within the previous 15 months (except patients who have never smoked) and have been given smoking cessation advice if appropriate.

✓ 90% should have had a record of their HBA1c within the previous 15 months. 50% of patients should have a level of ≤7.4% and 85% should have a level of ≤10%.

✓ 90% should have had retinal screening within the previous 15 months.

✓ 90% should have had a foot examination (including assessment of neuropathy and a peripheral pulse check) in the previous 15 months.

✓ 90% should have had a record of blood pressure (BP) within the previous 15 months. 55% should have a BP of ≤145/85 mmHg.

✓ 90% should have had a creatinine test and a microalbuminuria test within the previous 15 months. 70% of patients who test positive for microalbuminuria or proteinuria should be on an angiotensin converting enzyme (ACE) inhibitor or an angiotensin-II receptor blocker (ARB).

✓ 90% should have had a record of their total cholesterol within the previous 15 months. 60% should have a cholesterol of ≤5 mmol/l.

✓ 85% should have an annual influenza immunisation.

Is there evidence that improved glycaemic control leads to a reduction in complications?

There is significant evidence to confirm that meticulous glycaemic control can prevent or delay the onset of diabetic complications. The impact of these complications can also be greatly reduced if they are detected early and appropriately managed. Thus, regular surveillance for and early diagnosis of the complications of diabetes are very important. There are two very important studies regarding the importance of tight glycaemic control:

1. DCCT (Diabetes Control and Complications Trial)
(*N Engl J Med* 2000; **342**: 381–385)

✓ 1441 North American patients with type 1 diabetes.

✓ Randomised to intensive control or 'conventional' control.

✓ Patients receiving intensive insulin treatment had fewer microvascular complications.

✓ These benefits persisted with time.

✓ However, the improved glycaemic control was not completely advantageous to patients as it resulted in the need for more frequent home blood glucose testing and increased frequency of insulin injections.

✓ Many patients also gained weight and had an increased frequency of hypoglycaemic episodes.

✓ The group randomised to intensive control were telephoned regularly to remind them to be compliant.

 2. UKPDS (UK Prospective Diabetes Study)

This was a massive study involving over 5000 type 2 diabetic patients over a 20-year period, which resulted in numerous papers in the *Lancet* and the *BMJ*.

✓ In the arm of the study focusing on glycaemic control (*Lancet* 1998; **352**: 837–853), 5102 people with newly diagnosed type 2 diabetes were initially treated for 3 months with diet alone.

✓ Of the initial group, the 4209 patients who were asymptomatic and had fasting plasma glucose levels between 6 and 15 mmol/l were randomised to receive either intensive treatment with a sulphonylurea or with insulin (at the completion of the study this group had an average HBA1c of 7.0%) or conventional treatment (at the end of the study this group had an average HBA1c of 7.9%).

✓ The results showed that in the intensive group there was a 3.2% absolute risk reduction in the incidence of any diabetes-related adverse clinical endpoint (including diabetes-related deaths) over 10 years. Most of this benefit was due to a 2.7% absolute reduction in retinal photocoagulation. Further analysis showed a 2.4% absolute reduction in microvascular endpoints over 10 years. Although there were fewer macrovascular endpoints in the group receiving intensive treatment, this reduction failed to achieve statistical significance.

✓ Glycaemic control in both intensive and conventional groups deteriorated with time.

How often should we measure HbAlc?

According to NICE 2002 guidelines, HbAlc should be measured at 2- to 6-monthly intervals. The exact interval should depend on whether the patient has stable blood glucose levels, what their control is like and whether there have been any recent modifications to therapy.

HbAIc targets (NICE 2002)

The target HbAIc should be between 6.5% and 7.5%, based on the risk of macrovascular and microvascular complications. In general, people at significant risk of macrovascular complications should aim for an HbAIc of 6.5%, but higher targets are necessary for those at risk of iatrogenic hypoglycaemia.

The British Diabetic Association recommends that HbAIc be controlled to <6.5% for 'excellent control'. An HbAIc of >7.5% represents poor control.

Self-monitoring

According to NICE, self-monitoring should not be considered as a stand-alone intervention in type 2 diabetes. It recommends that self-monitoring should only be taught if there is a clear need for it or if there is a clear objective to be achieved – this should be agreed with the patient.

A recent editorial concluded that there is little evidence that self-monitoring significantly alters clinical outcomes in type 2 diabetes (*BMJ* 2004; **329**: 754–755). This is important because the costs involved in encouraging type 2 diabetics to self-monitor are huge – £90 million in 2001 (compared to £64 million spent on oral hypoglycaemics that year).

In a recent large study of non-insulin-treated type 2 diabetic patients, the performance and frequency of self-monitoring did not predict better control over a 3-year period (*Diabet Med* 2005; **22**: 900).

A multidisciplinary group of healthcare professionals published consensus advice on home blood glucose monitoring (*Diabet Primary Care* 2004; **6**: 8). The group agreed that monitoring was not required routinely in type 2 diabetes but suggested monitoring in special circumstances (during intercurrent illnesses, when oral hypoglycaemic treatment is changed, if systemic glucocorticoids are prescribed and if post-prandial hyperglycaemia occurs).

A recent good-quality systematic review following Cochrane methodology identified six relevant RCTs that fulfilled their predetermined quality standards (*Diabetes Care* 2005; **28**: 1510–1515). The overall effect in these trials was for self-monitoring to lower HbAIc by 0.39%, which the authors felt was a clinically significant benefit. There were a number of limitations in the studies reported.

Should there be a screening programme for type 2 diabetes?

The UKPDS study showed that about 50% of patients already had early signs of complications at the time of their diagnosis. Therefore, the question is raised of whether screening for diabetes should be introduced; if diabetes is diagnosed earlier, then theoretically, there would be a reduced incidence of complications. Certainly, it appears logical that patients at high risk are tested from time to time (eg South Asian and Afro-Caribbean patients and the obese).

Not everyone would agree with this view and various groups are lobbying the government to introduce screening (eg a 5-yearly OGTT for people over 40); however, this is not mentioned in the NSF, NICE or in the quality and outcomes framework of the new contract. There are issues of how the NHS would cope if screening were introduced and uncovered a huge previously undiagnosed cohort of type 2 diabetics (as it is likely to do) with all the attendant costs involved.

How important is treating hypertension in diabetic patients?

The UKPDS (BP-lowering arm) showed that any reduction in BP in type 2 diabetic patients reduces the risk of complications (*BMJ* 1998; **317**: 703–713). Intensive BP control is at least as (probably even more) important as intensive treatment of glucose levels in the reduction of complications in diabetic patients.

In the UKPDS BP study, 1148 people with hypertension and type 2 diabetes were randomised to a tight control arm (aiming at a BP of < 150/85 mmHg) or a less tight control arm (aiming at a BP of <180/105 mmHg). Over a median follow-up of 8.4 years, those in the tight control group had significant reductions in morbidity and mortality, with

✓ 24% relative reduction in all diabetes-related endpoints (NNT 6)

✓ 32% relative reduction in diabetes-related death (NNT 15)

✓ 44% relative reduction in fatal and non-fatal stroke (NNT 20)

✓ 37% relative reduction in developing microvascular complications (NNT 14)

✓ 21% relative reduction in MI.

The British Hypertension Society recommends a stricter target of 130/80 mmHg for diabetics, whereas the new contract has a less stringent target level of 145/85 mmHg.

The HOT study (*Lancet* 1998; **351**: 1755–1762) confirmed that tight BP control (130/80 mmHg) was more effective in diabetics than non-diabetics.

However, whether or not these targets are realistic is debatable; it has been estimated that the number of diabetics taking antihypertensive medication would need to double in order to meet even the target of 140/80 mmHg!

Should we give all diabetics ACE inhibitors?

A recent *Drug and Therapeutic Bulletin* (2005; **43(6)**: 41–45) looks at this issue in depth. Their conclusion was that the best evidence available suggests that it is the degree of BP control achieved that is important, not the class of antihypertensive used. They failed to find robust evidence for an 'ACE inhibitor effect' that exists independently of BP lowering. They point out that several of the largest hypertension studies (eg a meta-analysis involving 162,341 patients *Lancet* 2003; **362**: 1527–1235) have failed to find a difference in mortality rates between different antihypertensive regimes. The conclusion is that although ACE inhibitors are a reasonable choice when treating hypertension, they should not be prescribed routinely to all diabetics.

How do we treat diabetic nephropathy?

Tight BP control slows the progress of diabetic nephropathy. Patients with an elevated early morning urine albumin:creatinine ratio or with microalbuminuria on dipstick should be offered treatment with either an ACE inhibitor or an angiotensin receptor blocker.

The treatment of diabetic microalbuminuria and proteinuria with ACEIs or ARBs is now part of the quality and outcomes framework.

There is only limited evidence to support current guidelines that ACE inhibition is more beneficial than other BP-lowering regimes in treating microalbuminuria. The evidence is more robust for patients with frank proteinuria (*N Engl J Med* 2001; **345**: 851–860).

A recent systematic review concluded that ACEIs and ARBs have similar effects on renal outcomes but, unlike ACEIs, ARBs have not been shown to reduce mortality in patients with diabetic nephropathy (*BMJ* 2004; **329**: 828–831).

Therefore, ACEIs should be used as first-line treatment, and only patients who are intolerant of them should be changed to an ARB.

What is the evidence for statin use in diabetics?

Patients with type 2 diabetes should be considered as coronary heart disease (CHD) risk equivalents and dyslipidaemia should be a key therapeutic target, irrespective of baseline LDL cholesterol levels or age (*Circulation* 2004; **110**: 227). Four out of five deaths in patients with type 2 diabetes are caused by cardiovascular disease.

Diabetes has now been removed altogether from the Joint British Society risk charts, because it is assumed that almost all diabetics will qualify for treatment with a statin. Many experts feel that statins should be prescribed for the vast majority of patients with type 2 diabetes, irrespective of their baseline LDL cholesterol level (*Br J Diabetes Vasc Dis* 2005; **5**: 55).

The current recommendation in the GMS contract is to reduce total cholesterol to less than 5 mmol/l in all diabetic patients. However, the British Hypertension Society recommends that all type 2 diabetics over the age of 50 (or who have had their condition for at least 10 years) with a total cholesterol of >3.5 mmol/l should be considered to be CHD risk equivalents and should therefore be prescribed a statin. Other modifiable CHD risk factors such as smoking and obesity should also be addressed regularly.

The UKPDS ranked increased LDL cholesterol as the most important modifiable risk factor for CHD.

However, many diabetic patients are still not reaching current therapeutic lipid goals and so remain at an unacceptable level of risk (*JAMA* 2004; **291**: 335).

Results from the Heart Protection Study (HPS) showed that simvastatin could reduce the risk of MI, stroke or need for revascularisation in diabetic patients by a third, regardless of their cholesterol level (*Lancet* 2003; **361**: 2005). A meta-analysis of statin trials in diabetes concluded that the NNT to prevent one CHD event was only 13.8 over 4.9 years for secondary prevention and 34.5 over 4.3 years for primary prevention (*Ann Intern Med* 2004; **140**: 650).

The CARDS study involved over 2800 patients with type 2 diabetes and at least one other CHD risk factor (*Lancet* 2004; **364**: 685). It was stopped early when patients in the statin group showed significant reductions in MI, stroke, angina and revasculariation, even if they had normal LDL cholesterol levels (see Chapter 1, 'Hyperlipidaemia' section). However, although the CARDS study adds support to prescribing statins for all patients with type 2 diabetes, it is still recommended that the patient's individual risk and also preference should be considered when starting patients on long-term statin treatment.

What are the glitazones?

The thiazolidinediones or 'glitazones' are insulin sensitisers. They work by reducing the body's resistance to the action of insulin and enable a more efficient use of insulin. It should be noted that glycaemic control may not improve (or may even deteriorate if another oral hypoglycaemic has been withdrawn) initially with the introduction of one of these drugs – they tend to work best only after a few weeks.

Pioglitazone compared with rosiglitazone has been shown to be associated with significant improvements in triglycerides, HDL cholesterol and LDL cholesterol levels in patients with type 2 diabetes (*Diabetes Care* 2005; **28**: 1547).

The glitazones are expensive and NICE issued guidance in 2003 suggesting that the use of these drugs should be limited to patients who cannot tolerate metformin and a sulphonylurea in combination, either because of an intolerance or a contraindication.

PROactive study (*Lancet* 2005; **366**: 1279–1289)

✓ Looked at the effect of adding pioglitazone to existing oral hypoglycaemic therapy.

✓ 5238 patients with type 2 diabetes who had evidence of macrovascular disease.

✓ The mean follow-up time was for 34.5 months.

✓ The primary endpoint was the composite of all-cause mortality, non-fatal myocardial infarction, stroke, acute coronary syndrome, intervention in the coronary or leg arteries, and amputation above the ankle.

✓ 514 of 2605 patients in the pioglitazone group and 572 of 2633 patients in the placebo group had at least one event in the primary composite endpoint (2.2% absolute risk reduction; NNT 46). This did not reach statistical significance.

✓ The authors claim that their study is the first to ever show that taking oral hypoglycaemics can prevent macrovascular events.

However, the results of this long-awaited trial have actually raised more questions than answers about the role of glitazones for diabetics. There was an increased incidence of heart failure in patients taking pioglitazone. In addition, some critics have commented that the cardiovascular benefits of pioglitazone over placebo were unlikely to have been demonstrated had all patients received statins (only 43% of patients were on statins at the start of the study).

A recent article challenges the interpretation of the PROactive study, stating that this interpretation is based on secondary outcomes (the primary outcome remained neutral), and also explains why the conclusions presented may be statistically unsound and unsafe (*BMJ* 2005; **331**: 836).

What about the meglitinides?

Repaglinide and nateglinide stimulate insulin secretion. Both have a rapid onset of action and a short-lasting effect. They are licensed for combination therapy with metformin in type 2 diabetes and repaglinide is also licensed as monotherapy. These drugs are effective in reducing post-prandial glucose concentrations; however, it is not yet known whether this effect is clinically beneficial in terms of cardiovascular outcomes.

Inhaled insulin

✓ 'Exubera®' has been developed by Pfizer.

✓ It is likely to be licensed in 2006.

✓ Short-acting.

✓ 20% absorbed.

✓ Unsuitable for smokers, recent ex-smokers, patients with significant lung disease, women who may become pregnant and children.

✓ Improved patient satisfaction compared to subcutaneous insulin.

✓ Large device, five steps per inhalation; several inhalations per meal necessary.

What does all this mean for patients?

It is well known that in practice it is very difficult to maintain optimal glycaemic and BP control, even with multiple drug combinations. Even under the stringent conditions of the ASCOT trial, only 32% of diabetic patients achieved their target BP of 130/80 mmHg. The polypharmacy involved is a daunting prospect for any diabetic patient. If HbA1c quality and outcomes framework targets are to be achieved, many more diabetics are going to need to be started on insulin.

The compliance of diabetic patients is poorer than expected – one study (*Diabet Med* 2002; **19**: 279–284) collected anonymous information on prescriptions from diabetic patients in Dundee, which showed that only one-third of patients comply with single medications and about one-tenth comply with two medications!

The future of diabetes care in the UK will be challenging to GPs. Although clear therapeutic goals have been defined, doctors may need to negotiate realistic goals with individual patients regarding their optimal treatment.

Impaired glucose tolerance (IGT)

Impaired glucose tolerance (IGT; defined as a fasting plasma glucose of <7 mmol/l with a 2-h OGTT value of 7.8–11.1 mmol/l) is a common condition affecting up to 17% of people aged 40–65 in the UK.

People with impaired glucose tolerance have increased cardiovascular mortality; the Whitehall study (*Lancet* 1980; **1**: 1373–1376) showed that it doubled the risk of death from CHD among middle-aged male civil servants.

Approximately 50% of patients with IGT will develop type 2 diabetes over a 10-year period. Although their risk of cardiovascular disease is high, these patients do not appear to be at greater risk of microvascular disease.

How can we stop people with IGT from developing diabetes?

Interventions that have been shown to be of benefit include exercise and weight loss. In one very interesting study, the Diabetes Prevention Program Research Group/Outcome Study, over 3000 patients with impaired fasting glucose or glucose intolerance were randomised to placebo, metformin or an 'intensive lifestyle modification program' (involving at least 150 minutes of exercise per week and a weight-reducing diet) (*N Engl J Med* 2002; **346**: 393–403). Patients were followed-up for just under 3 years. The most effective intervention was found to be lifestyle intervention – approximately seven people needed to be treated for one year to prevent one case of diabetes, compared to 14 patients on metformin. This NNT is certainly more impressive than for most drugs.

The metabolic syndrome

Insulin resistance is thought to be the aetiological factor behind the 'metabolic syndrome' which consists of hypertension, high triglycerides, low HDL and central obesity. At least 20% of the adult population and about 40% of adults aged over 60 years have metabolic syndrome (*Diabetes Care* 2004; **27**: 2444). There are different definitions of the metabolic syndrome.

The International Diabetes Federation definition is as follows:

✓ Waist circumference ≥80 cm in women or 94 cm in men plus any two of the following four factors:

- Triglycerides ≥1.7 mmol/l

- HDL <1.03 mmol/l in men or 1.29 mmol/l in women

- BP >130/85 mmHg

- Fasting glucose ≥5.6 mmol/l.

Metabolic syndrome is associated with increased risk of type 2 diabetes (*Diabetes Care* 2004; **27**: 2676) and also cardiovascular disease (*Circulation* 2004; **110**: 1251).

The addition of a glitazone for type 2 diabetic subjects with metabolic syndrome has been shown to be associated to a reduction in insulin resistance (*Diabetes Res Clin Pract* 2005; **69**: 5).

Rosiglitazone plus metformin significantly improved long-term control of insulin-resistance-related parameters compared with glimepiride plus metformin in a recent study (*J Int Med Res* 2005; **33**: 284).

One study showed, rather worryingly, that South Asian children aged 8–11 years in the UK already had higher levels of insulin and insulin resistance than white children (*BMJ* 2002; **324**: 635–638). Insulin resistance is certainly a huge problem in the South Asian population, and may help to explain why the mortality rate from CHD in this group is 40–50% higher than in their Caucasian counterparts.

USEFUL WEBSITES

www.diabetes.org.uk – Diabetes UK

www.audit-commission.gov.uk – Audit
Commission report

www.nsc.nhs.uk – National Screening Committee
website – evaluation

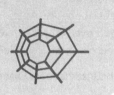

SUMMARY POINTS

✓ Incidence of diabetes is increasing

✓ All cardiovascular risk factors need to be addressed

✓ Targets are often difficult to reach

✓ Regular HbA1c testing may be as effective as
home monitoring

✓ Meticulous glycaemic control can reduce
complications

✓ Screening for diabetes is not cost-effective

CHAPTER 3:
RESPIRATORY DISEASES

CHAPTER 3: RESPIRATORY DISEASES

Asthma

Asthma affects approximately 8 million people in the UK at some stage in their lives. It has been estimated to cost the NHS £850 million a year, with half the costs arising as a result of acute asthma attacks. Over 18 million working days are lost to asthma each year. The ultimate goal for the management of asthma is to help patients lead a normal life, free from symptoms and with no limitations on activities.

Many asthmatic patients misunderstand the severity of their condition. A survey of mild-to-moderate asthma patients revealed that although 91% of them felt that their asthma was well controlled, 66% had symptoms at least twice a week. Only a third of patients were satisfied with their current asthma care (*Primary Care Resp J* 2004; **13**: 28).

Diagnosis

This is based on variability of peak flow or spirometry.

- ✓ ≥20% variability in peak expiratory flow rate (PEFR, ≥60 l/min) for 3 days in a week for at least 2 weeks.

- ✓ ≥20% improvement in PEFR 10 min after high-dose beta-agonist (through spacer) (or 15%/200 ml improvement in forced expiratory volume in 1 s, FEV_1).

- ✓ ≥20% improvement in PEFR after 14 days of prednisolone (30 mg).

British Thoracic Society (BTS) guidelines – key points

The BTS guidelines were revised in 2003 and then further updated in 2004.

Points of note include:

✓ Inhaled steroids (at a dose of 400 micrograms/day of beclometasone in adults or 200 micrograms/day in children) should be considered if a patient has had an exacerbation of their asthma in the past 2 years **or** if they are symptomatic, needing a beta-agonist at least 3 times a week **or** if they are symptomatic at least 1 night per week. Exercise-induced asthma is often (but not always) a sign of poor control.

✓ Adults who are considered to require inhaled steroids should initially be started off on a moderate dose, eg 400–800 micrograms beclometasone.

✓ Steroids taken twice daily are slightly more effective than once-daily steroids. However, once good control is established, once-a-day inhaled steroids at the same total dose can be considered. This may have the advantage of improving compliance (*Primary Care Resp J* 2005; **14**: 88–98).

✓ Long-acting beta-agonists are now used at step 3 instead of increasing the inhaled corticosteroid dose to beyond 800 micrograms per day. The MIASMA systematic analysis (*BMJ* 2000; **320**: 1368–1373) provided proof that salmeterol added to low or moderate doses of inhaled corticosteroids was more effective at increasing FEV_1 and reducing symptoms than higher doses of inhaled steroids.

✓ The BTS no longer recommends that patients should double their dose of inhaled steroid during an asthma exacerbation, due to lack of evidence of efficacy (*Thorax* 2004; **59**: 550–556; *Lancet* 2004; **363**: 271–275). However, in practice, many patients feel that there is benefit in doing this. Interestingly, asthma self-management plans that include doubling the dose of inhaled steroid when the patient deteriorates have been shown to improve asthma control. Some experts recommend that the patient should actually treble or quadruple their inhaled steroid for up to two weeks during an exacerbation, starting in the 'window period' when their symptoms first begin to show signs of deterioration.

General Medical Services (GMS) contract and asthma

To achieve maximum quality points, the following standards need to be met:

✓ The practice must have an up to date register of asthmatic patients (excluding those who have not been prescribed asthma-related drugs in the past year).

✓ 70% of adults and children >8 years old should have had their diagnosis confirmed by serial peak flows or spirometry.

✓ 70% of patients >14 years need to have an up to date record of their smoking status within the previous 15 months (the exception being adults who have never smoked, who only need to have their status recorded once).

✓ 70% of asthmatics who smoke should have been offered smoking cessation advice within the previous 15 months.

✓ 70% of asthmatics should have had an annual review within the previous 15 months.

✓ 70% of asthmatics >16 years old should have an annual influenza vaccination.

How safe are inhaled steroids?

The amount of inhaled steroid absorbed in the body is very low, but systemic side-effects can occur, eg osteoporosis, growth retardation and symptoms of adrenal suppression. Side-effects are unlikely with low-dose inhaled steroids (<400 micrograms beclometasone/day in children and <800 micrograms/day in adults). All children receiving inhaled steroids should have their height measured regularly, and any children needing high maintenance doses are best supervised by a paediatrician. Children with a viral-associated wheeze should not usually be prescribed inhaled steroids.

The Cochrane Airways Group has reviewed six randomised controlled trials looking at patients with asthma or chronic obstructive pulmonary disease (COPD) who were on inhaled steroids. No significant rise in bone turnover was found in any of the studies up to 3 years after steroids were first prescribed, provided they had been given at recommended BTS levels. However, one study found that therapeutic doses of inhaled steroids can significantly lower bone mineral density (BMD) as measured in the spine and femur in adults on regular treatment for at least 6 years (*Lancet* 2000; **1385**: 1399).

The 2003 BTS guidelines advocate introducing long-acting beta-2-agonists before increasing the dose of inhaled steroids above 800 micrograms per day.

Decreasing the dose of inhaled steroids

The most important safeguard for patients is to have their asthma reviewed regularly, and the dose of inhaled steroid stepped down once control of symptoms is achieved. Current BTS guidelines state that patients should be on the lowest effective dose of inhaled steroids and a reduction in the dose should be considered every 3 months for stable patients; each time by 25–50%.

What is the best way to review asthmatics?

Although included in the quality and outcomes framework of the new contract, it is very difficult to persuade asthmatics to attend for regular review. This is partly because it is difficult for many asthmatics to attend during surgery hours and partly because many do not consider themselves to have a chronic disease. More and more GPs are now using telephone reviews to help combat this problem, using the Royal College of Physicians morbidity index questions (see below); patients who answer yes to any one of these three questions should be invited to attend for a review. There is some evidence that this strategy is cost-effective and saves time.

Important trials

Predicting exacerbations in asthma (*J Gen Intern Med* 2004; **19**: 237–242)

In terms of monitoring patients with asthma, there is increasing evidence that asking about quality of life indicators is better than measuring peak flow in terms of predicting an exacerbation. Questions recommended by the Royal College of Physicians are:

- ✓ Have you had your usual asthma symptoms during the day?
- ✓ Have you had any difficulty in sleeping because of your asthma?
- ✓ Has your asthma interfered with your usual activities?

In this study, quality of life indicators were found to be as good as PEFR at predicting asthma exacerbations.

- ✓ This study was set in 36 pharmacies and involved 660 asthmatic patients.

✓ Patients were randomised to receive 'usual care' or a PEFR meter.

✓ Quality of life indicators were assessed at 0, 6 and 12 months.

✓ Patients were phoned monthly to obtain information about PEFR readings and to ask whether they had suffered from an exacerbation in the past month.

✓ Quality of life indicators were found to be independent predictors of exacerbation at 4 months and 12 months.

IMPACT trial; does mild, persistent asthma require regular treatment? (*N Engl J Med* 2005; **352**: 1519–1524)

This trial compared regular inhaled corticosteroid (ICS) therapy (with 200 micrograms budesonide bd) with no regular treatment or with oral zafirlukast in patients with mild asthma. The conclusion was that it is possible to treat mild, persistent asthma with short, intermittent courses of inhaled or oral steroids taken only when symptoms worsen.

✓ 225 non-smoking adults with mild asthma (FEV_1 >70% predicted, less than daily use of bronchodilators, night time waking less than once a week) were randomised to one of three treatment arms: regular budesonide, regular oral zafirlukast or no regular treatment.

✓ Primary outcome was morning peak flow.

✓ Patients were asked to take budesonide 800 micrograms bd for 10 days or oral prednisolone (0.5mg/kg body wt per day) for 5 days if their asthma symptoms worsened.

✓ Patients were given a written summary of this plan.

✓ The three treatments produced similar increases in morning PEF and there were similar rates of asthma exacerbations, even though the placebo group only took budesonide for an average of 0.5 weeks per year.

✓ Oral zafirlukast did not differ from placebo.

✓ Regular inhaled budesonide resulted in greater improvements in pre-bronchodilator FEV_1, bronchial reactivity, scores for asthma and symptom-free days (26 additional days per year), but not in post-bronchodilator FEV_1, morning PEFR or in quality of life scores.

Asthmatic smokers are resistant to inhaled steroids (*Thorax* 2005; **60**: 282–287)

✓ Multicentre randomised trial.

✓ Smokers given 400 micrograms beclometasone showed little improvement in markers of asthma severity compared to the expected improvement in non-smokers and had 6 times as many exacerbations over the follow-up period of 12 weeks.

✓ Higher doses of inhaled steroids (2000 micrograms daily) seemed to be more effective; at this dose, smokers did improve in terms of lung function tests and also reduced their usage of short-acting bronchodilators. However, non-smokers still had better results.

Review of occupational asthma (*Br J Gen Prac* 2004; **54**: 731–733)

✓ Occupational asthma is the most frequently reported occupational respiratory disease in the UK.

✓ 1500–3000 people develop occupational asthma per year as a direct result of environmental factors in the work place.

✓ All newly diagnosed adults with asthma should be asked about their occupation and whether their symptoms are worse at work.

✓ People in the following occupations are at particular risk: painters, bakers, nurses and people who work with animals.

✓ These patients should be referred to an occupational health physician.

Systematic review on aspirin induced asthma (*BMJ* 2004; **328**: 434)

Aspirin-induced asthma is a distinct clinical syndrome affecting some asthmatic patients. It is characterised by the onset of asthma 30 min to 3 h after the ingestion of aspirin.

This paper found that 21% of asthmatics have evidence of an asthmatic response after ingestion of aspirin. Almost all these patients displayed cross-sensitivity to NSAIDs (98% to ibuprofen and 100% to naproxen) and 7% were also sensitive to paracetamol.

Cochrane review on inhaled beta-2 agonists for treating non-specific chronic cough in children (*Cochrane Library* 2005, Issue 3)

All RCTs including children >2 who were given inhaled beta-2 agonists for chronic cough (lasting >3/52).

✓ In children presenting with chronic cough, there was no benefit of salbutamol over placebo.

✓ The existence of cough-variant asthma is controversial.

Which other drugs are available to treat asthma?

Leukotriene receptor antagonists are a class of oral asthma therapies that have anti-inflammatory and bronchodilator properties. Currently they seem to be best used as add-ons to low- or high-dose inhaled steroids where control of persistent asthma symptoms has not been achieved, or instead of steroids for children under 5 years.

A systematic review examined the evidence for the efficacy and glucocorticoid-sparing effect of oral antileukotrienes in asthmatic patients (*BMJ* 2002; **324**: 1545–1548). This showed that these drugs may modestly improve the control of asthma compared to glucocorticoids alone. A more recent trial has shown that adding montelukast to the treatment regimes of asthma patients whose symptoms were uncontrolled with fluticasone provided equivalent control to adding salmeterol (*BMJ* 2003; **327**: 891–895).

There is still little evidence, however, to support the use of leukotriene receptor antagonists (LTRAs) as a substitute for inhaled glucocorticoids. A systematic review (*BMJ* 2003; **326**: 621) compared LTRAs to inhaled steroids and found that inhaled steroids were more effective (at a dosage equivalent to 400 micrograms beclometasone per day), with a 60% lower risk of exacerbation.

Do self-management plans have a role in asthma management?

Asthma lends itself to the use of guided self-management plans based on the BTS guidelines. There is plenty of evidence which shows that the use of self-management plans for asthma can lead to a reduction in hospitalisation rates and, time off work, and improvement in symptom control. However, many asthmatic patients do not regard their condition as a chronic disease that needs regular monitoring and therapeutic adjustments, but instead prefer to manage it as an intermittent acute disorder.

Revisions to the evidence-based BTS/SIGN guidelines means that the patient is placed at the centre of asthma management. Asthmatic patients should be trained to manage their own treatment by using personal asthma action plans (PAAPs). A written PAAP aids detection of deteriorating asthma control and offers straightforward advice in terms of appropriate drug treatment. Such plans must be devised on an individual basis and formulated according to personal best peak expiratory flow, symptoms, or both (*Thorax* 2004; **59**: 94). However, implementation of PAAPs and education in asthma self-management remains poor (*Thorax* 2004; **59**: 87).

Key components of a written asthma action plan

✓ Peak expiratory flow based on personal best values and not predicted values.

✓ Two to four levels of intervention in terms of symptoms or lung function.

✓ Advice as to when to use oral corticosteroids.

What is the association between asthma and allergic rhinitis?

Between 30% and 90% of asthmatics also have hayfever and an exacerbation of allergic rhinitis can lead to an exacerbation in asthma symptoms (*Current Med Res Opin* 2004; **20**: 1549–1558). It is likely that, in the future, more emphasis will be placed on the importance of treating both conditions concomitantly.

New BTS guidelines for asthma (2003)

Step 1 Inhaled short-acting beta-2-agonist as required. If more than 3 times a week on average, go to step 2.

Step 2 Add inhaled steroid 200–800 micrograms/day. Start at dose of inhaled steroid appropriate to severity of disease. In children <5, a leukotriene receptor antagonist (LRA) could be considered instead of the steroid. In children aged 5–12 years, add inhaled steroid to a maximum of 400 micrograms/day.

Step 3 Add long-acting beta–2-agonist (LABA) or consider LRA in children < 5 years.

✓ If inadequate response, continue LABA, but increase inhaled steroid dose to 800 micrograms per day (400 micrograms in children aged 5–12).

✓ If no response to LABA, stop LABA and increase inhaled steroids to 800 micrograms/day (400 micrograms in children). If control still inadequate, consider LRAs/ theophylline in adults and children.

✓ Refer children under 2 at this stage or at stage 4 if between 2 and 5 years of age.

Step 4 Consider trials of:

✓ Increasing inhaled steroids up to 2000 micrograms/day (800 micrograms in children aged 5–12 years).

✓ Addition of a fourth drug, eg LRA, SR theophylline, beta-2-agonist tablet.

Step 5 Daily steroid tablet in lowest dose providing adequate control, whilst maintaining high-dose inhaled steroid at 2000 micrograms/day (or 800 micrograms in children aged 5–12). Consider referral in most adults and all children <12.

USEFUL WEBSITES

www.gpiag.org – GPs in asthma group

www.brit-thoracic.org.uk – British Thoracic Society

www.asthma.org.uk – National Asthma Campaign

SUMMARY POINTS FOR ASTHMA

✓ Essential to learn BTS guidelines

✓ Many asthmatic patients are still not adequately controlled

✓ Patients should be central to their management

✓ Patient expectations of asthma control are very low

Chronic obstructive pulmonary disease

Chronic obstructive pulmonary disease (COPD) is the fourth leading cause of death worldwide and causes over 30,000 deaths a year in the UK (*Lancet* 2004; **364**: 564). It is both under-diagnosed and under-recognised. Many people with COPD do not consult their GP or do not reveal all their symptoms unless specifically asked (*Prim Care Resp J* 2002; **11**: S12).

Whereas COPD was considered to have few therapeutic options previously, it is now considered treatable as there has been increasing evidence supporting both pharmacological and non-pharmacological treatments (*BMJ* 2004; **329**: 361).

Diagnosis

Airflow obstruction is defined as FEV_1/FVC <0.7 after using a bronchodilator, or FEV_1 <80% of the predicted value.

If the FEV_1 is between 50% and 80% of predicted, the disease is considered to be 'mild'.

An FEV_1 of between 30% and 50% signifies moderate disease.

An FEV_1 of <30% of the predicted value signifies severe disease.

	COPD	Asthma
FEV_1	Always reduced (FEV_1/FVC <70%)	Variable
Diurnal variation	Minimal	Morning dip
Increase in FEV_1 post bronchodilator	<200 ml	>500 ml (≥20%)
Response to steroid trial	Partial response in 10–20%	Good

Table: COPD vs asthma

NICE guidelines

<table>
<tr><td rowspan="5" style="writing-mode: vertical-lr">STOP THERAPY IF INEFFECTIVE</td><td>• Use short-acting bronchodilator prn (beta-2-agonist or anticholinergic)</td></tr>
<tr><td>• If still syptomatic try combined therapy with a short-acting beta-2-agonist and a short-acting anticholinergic</td></tr>
<tr><td>• If still syptomatic use a long-acting bronchodilator (beta$_2$-agonist or anticholinergic)</td></tr>
<tr><td>• In moderate or severe chronic obstructive pulmonary disease: if still symptomatic consider a trial of a combination of a long-acting beta$_2$-agonist and inhaled corticosteroid. Discontinue if no benefit after 4 weeks</td></tr>
<tr><td>• If still symptomatic consider adding theophylline</td></tr>
<tr><td colspan="2">• Offer pulmonary rehabilitation to all patients who consider themselves functionally disabled (usually MRC grade 3 and above)</td></tr>
<tr><td colspan="2">• Consider referral for surgery: bullectomy, lung volume reduction surgery, transplantation</td></tr>
</table>

NICE updated their guidance on COPD in 2004 (see below for algorithm).

Important points of note are:

✓ Inhaled corticosteroids (ICS) can now be prescribed for patients with moderate to severe COPD (ie with an FEV$_1$ of ≤50%) who have had more than two exacerbations in the preceding year or whose symptoms are not controlled by a combination of short- and long-acting bronchodilators. A 'steroid trial' is no longer necessary and inhaled steroids can be continued if there is found to be clinical benefit after 4 weeks; formal retesting with spirometry is no longer required. There is evidence that ICS reduce the rate of exacerbations (*Am J Med* 2002; **113**: 59–65).

✓ Mucolytics can be used for patients with a chronic, productive cough. However, there is no evidence that they improve lung function or reduce exacerbation rates (*Lancet* 2005; **365**: 1552–1560).

✓ If short-acting bronchodilators are insufficient to control symptoms, there is a choice between using a long-acting beta-2-agonist or a long-acting anticholinergic (tiotropium).

✓ Stopping smoking is the most effective intervention in terms of stopping decline of respiratory function, although it does not restore lost function.

✓ The Royal College of Physicians have recommended that long-term oxygen therapy should be considered in severe cases of COPD where the PaO_2 <7.3 kPa, or moderate cases (PaO_2 7.3–8 kPa) in the presence of secondary polycythaemia, nocturnal hypoxaemia, peripheral oedema or pulmonary hypertension. Oxygen therapy only increases survival if used for >15 h per day.

What evidence is there for inhaled steroids?

This is quite controversial. Some RCTs have shown that there is no significant difference between inhaled steroids and placebo in lung function (ie FEV_1) over 10 days to 10 weeks. Current guidelines recommend that inhaled steroids should be used in patients with an FEV_1 of less than 50% predicted or with two or more exacerbations a year. However, in practice, steroids are prescribed for far more COPD patients – it has been estimated that 80% of patients with COPD received them in primary care.

✓ However, a systematic review found that long-term steroids reduce the frequency of exacerbations (*Am J Med* 2002; **2002**: 59–65).

✓ The ISOLDE study was a large RCT, which found that inhaled fluticasone reduced the median exacerbation rate in patients with severe COPD by 25% (*BMJ* 2000; **320**: 1297–1303).

✓ The TRISTAN study group showed that treatment of COPD with combined fluticasone and salmeterol significantly increased FEV_1 after 12 months of treatment: more than either drug used individually (*Lancet* 2003; **361**: 449–456).

✓ A recent analysis has shown that mortality in COPD may be cut by 27% with the use of inhaled corticosteroids (*Thorax* 2005:992-7).

The *Drug and Therapeutics Bulletin* concurs with NICE and suggests that a trial of inhaled steroids should be reserved for patients who have an FEV_1 of <50% and who have frequent exacerbations, or those who have had a spirometric response.

Which is better – inhaled anticholinergics or beta-2-agonists?

Although long-acting bronchodilators have been an important advance for the management of COPD, these drugs do not deal with the underlying inflammatory process (*Eur Respir J* 2005; **25**: 1084).

Compared with salmeterol twice daily, the long-acting anticholinergic drug tiotropium provides superior bronchodilation for 24 h (*Chest* 2004; **125**: 249). This study also showed that long-acting bronchodilators improve patient-centred outcomes such as exercise capacity, dyspnoea and health-related quality of life.

There is currently insufficient evidence to recommend fixed-dose LABA/steroid combination therapy (ie seretide) over variable-dose combined therapy (ie symbicort) or vice versa. Trials sponsored by the individual drug companies have produced conflicting results (usually in favour of the product manufactured by that particular drug company!).

Hospital at home for patients with an acute exacerbation of COPD (*BMJ* 2004; **329**: 315–318)

- ✓ Systematic review examining 7 trials including 754 patients.

- ✓ Primary endpoint was mortality and readmission to hospital.

- ✓ No significant difference between the groups in the primary endpoint.

- ✓ Concluded that hospital at home schemes can be safely used to care for patients with acute exacerbations of COPD who would be otherwise admitted to hospital, which is much cheaper.

What is the evidence for nurse-led management of patients with COPD? Systematic review (*BMJ* 2005; **331**: 485–488)

- ✓ Nine RCTs.

- ✓ Two studies looked at brief interventions (1 month); neither found any benefit.

- ✓ Meta-analysis of interventions lasting a year failed to detect any influence on mortality at 9- to 12-months follow-up.

- ✓ There was no improvement in patients' health-related quality of life scores, psychological wellbeing, disability or pulmonary function with long-term interventions.

- ✓ There is very little evidence to support widespread implementation of nurse-led management interventions for COPD.

Exercise programmes and rehabilitation

A review of the effects of exercise in mild to moderate COPD showed improved exercise tolerance and health status (*BJGP* 2002; **52**: 574). A meta-analysis concluded that pulmonary rehabilitation (lasting at least 4 weeks) comprising graded exercise training, education and psychological/behavioural therapy (including smoking cessation advice) reduces breathlessness and increases quality of life (*Lancet* 1996; **348**: 1115–1119). NICE recommends that all patients with COPD who consider themselves to be 'functionally disabled' should be referred for pulmonary rehabilitation.

COPD causes a great deal of social and psychological morbidity; in advanced COPD, 80% of patients are housebound. There is a high prevalence of anxiety and depression among patients with chronic breathing disorders (*Chest* 2005; **127**: 1205). According to this study, 65% screened positive for depression and anxiety, 10% for anxiety only and 5% for depression only.

GMS Contract and COPD

The New Contract correctly identifies COPD as a significant problem in primary care. It places emphasis on the detection of airflow obstruction by spirometry – which may be difficult for some practices. Bronchodilator reversibility testing is also required although there is some debate as to whether or not this is necessary clinically.

To achieve maximum quality points, the following standards must be met:

- ✓ The practice must have a register of COPD patients.

- ✓ 90% of patients should have had their diagnosis confirmed by spirometry, including reversibility testing.

- ✓ 90% of COPD patients should have had a record of their smoking status within the previous 15 months.

- ✓ 90% of smokers should have received smoking cessation advice within the previous 15 months.

- ✓ 70% of patients should have had their FEV_1 recorded within the previous 27 months.

- ✓ 90% of patients should have had their inhaler technique checked in the previous 2 years.

- ✓ 85% should receive an influenza immunisation.

SUMMARY POINTS

✓ The NICE guidelines provide evidence-based advice

✓ Smoking cessation advice is vital

✓ Pulmonary rehabilitation is very effective

✓ Long-term oxygen therapy improves survival

✓ COPD is often associated with depression

USEFUL WEBSITES

www.brit-thoracic.org.uk – British Thoracic Society

www.nice.org.uk – NICE

www.goldcopd.com – WHO Global Initiative for Chronic Obstructive Lung Disease

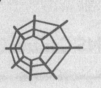

Smoking cessation

Around one in four adults smoke, with much higher levels in deprived sections of society. Many young people smoke; approximately 1% of 11-year-olds smoke regularly. This figure rises to 26% for girls and 21% for boys aged 15. Smoking is the single most important cause of preventable illness and premature death in the UK, and leads to direct medical costs of £1.7b each year (about 0.16% of the gross domestic product) (*BMJ* 2004; **328**: 947).

Giving up permanently is difficult; although two-thirds of smokers want to quit, and about one-third try each year, only 2% actually succeed. One study found that 16% of English smokers are 'hardcore' – defined as having had less than a day without cigarettes in the past 5 years, no desire to quit and no intention to quit (*BMJ* 2003; **326**: 1061). They are more likely to be older and from more socioeconomically deprived backgrounds. In addition they are more likely to dismiss any effects of smoking on their health.

On average, 70% of smokers consult their GP each year, so primary care teams need to be involved with smoking cessation programmes.

In December 2000, Thorax published updated guidelines for tackling cigarette dependence (*Thorax* 2000; **55**: 987–999). They recognise that GPs have a pivotal role if the NHS is to deliver a noticeable drop in smoking rates. These guidelines are based on strong evidence from randomised trials supplemented by studies examining what can be achieved in routine clinical practice. There has since been a systematic review published, which is discussed below (*Tob Control* 2003; **12**: 21–27).

What are the advantages of stopping smoking?

There are obviously huge benefits from stopping smoking; 25% of smokers will die prematurely as a direct result of their habit.

The follow-up results of the landmark prospective study on smoking and lung cancer in the 1950s by Richard Doll *et al*. have now been published (*BMJ* 2004; **328**: 1519–1533). This cohort of >34,000 British male doctors were originally questioned about their smoking habits in 1951 and periodically thereafter. Cause specific mortality was monitored for 50 years.

- ✓ Unlike in non-smokers, longevity did not continue to improve in those who continued smoking.

- ✓ Among those born around 1920, cigarette smoking tripled age-specific mortality.

- ✓ Stopping at 50 years of age halved the hazard.

- ✓ Stopping at 30 years of age avoided almost all the hazard.

- ✓ Stopping at age 60, 50, 40 or 30 gains, respectively, approximately 3, 6, 9, or 10 years of life expectancy.

- ✓ Stopping smoking before middle age avoids more than 90% of the risk attributable to tobacco. Widespread cessation of smoking in the UK has already halved the lung cancer mortality that would have been expected if former smokers had continued to smoke.

Although there is no doubt that smoking cessation reduces decline in lung function, this benefit may be offset to some extent by weight gain (*Lancet* 2005; **365**: 1629–1635). The authors of this study looked at data from a European population-based survey which included 6654 people who had their lung function measured in 1991–1993 and again in 1998–2002. Overall, both men and women lost 0.8% of their lung function each year and this decline was fastest in smokers. Unfortunately, people who quit between the two surveys put on the most weight and each kilogram of weight gain was found to diminish the benefit of quitting by 38% in men and 17% in women over the 9-year follow-up period. Although there was still benefit from quitting smoking, this study highlights the importance of helping such patients to control their food intake.

How effective are smoking cessation treatments?

Smoking cessation results in a 36% reduction in relative risk of mortality (*BMJ* 2005; **12**: 37). Nicotine replacement therapy (NRT) products approximately double the chance of long-term abstinence. Though services aimed at smoking cessation have made extensive use of the stage-based approach, a systematic review has shown that only limited evidence exists for its effectiveness (*BMJ* 2003; **326**: 1175). One observational study has shown that current NHS smoking cessation services are unlikely to be reducing the prevalence of smoking by more than 0.1–0.3% a year (*BMJ* 2005; **330**: 760).

Clinics to help people stop smoking have led to an increased number of GPs recording whether patients smoke and referring them for assistance to quit (*Public Health* 2005; **119**: 262).

The NHS Centre for Reviews and Dissemination (University of York) has produced a systematic review of smoking cessation treatments. The results show that both NRT and bupropion are cost-effective treatments in terms of cost per life-year saved.

Quit smoking schemes (*Ann Intern Med* 2005: **142**: 233–239)

✓ US and Canadian study.

✓ 5887 patients in a 10-week programme that included discussions with a doctor, group sessions on behavioural modification and NRT.

✓ Participants were followed up for 14.5 years, and compared to usual care controls.

✓ After 5 years, 21.7% of the treatment group had stopped smoking compared to 5.4% of controls. At the end of follow-up, all-cause mortality was 8.83/1000 compared to 10.38/1000 in controls.

✓ Smoking cessation schemes can have a substantial effect on long-term mortality.

Passive smoking

Exposure at work might account for 20% of all deaths from passive smoking in the 20- to 64-year age group, and for up to 50% of such deaths among people who work in the hospitality industry (*BMJ* 2005; **330**: 812–815). Smoking has now been banned in public places in Ireland, and England and Wales may follow suit in the future.

Nicotine replacement therapy (NRT)

This treatment aims to replace the nicotine obtained from cigarettes, thus reducing withdrawal symptoms when stopping smoking. Nicotine replacement is available as chewing gum, transdermal patch, nasal spray, inhaler, sublingual tablet and lozenge. A Cochrane review of over 90 trials found that nicotine replacement helps people to stop smoking. Overall, it increases the chances of quitting by about 1.5–2 times, whatever the level of additional support and encouragement.

There is little direct evidence that one nicotine product is more effective than another. Thus, the decision about which product to use should be guided by individual preferences. Combining a patch with other forms of NRT may be more effective than a patch alone and appears to have a good safety profile. A systematic review found that over-the-counter NRT works as well as prescribed NRT, even if the prescription is combined with a behavioural programme (*Tob Control* 2003; **12**: 21–27).

What is bupropion (Zyban®)?

This was initially developed as an antidepressant. One hypothesis of its mode of action is that it works by increasing levels of dopamine and noradrenaline in the brain, thereby counteracting the reductions in these chemicals that result from nicotine withdrawal. The efficacy of bupropion as an aid to smoking cessation has been investigated in two randomised, double-blinded, placebo-controlled trials (*N Engl J Med* 1997; **337**: 1195–1202 and *N Engl J Med* 1999; **340**: 685–691). These patients received regular counselling sessions in addition to bupropion. Results have indicated that up to 30% of smokers succeed with bupropion and that these results are sustained over a year.

Bupropion is relatively well tolerated; contraindications to its use include epilepsy, pregnancy and concomitant antidepressants. The risk of fits has been estimated at about 1 in 1000 people, which is actually the same risk as for amitriptyline and imipramine. It may also increase the risk of fits through interactions with other drugs that lower the seizure threshold, including antipsychotics, antidepressants, systemic steroids, antimalarial drugs and theophylline. It has recently been shown that bupropion does not appear to increase the risk of sudden death, contrary to previous concerns (*Thorax* 2005; **60**: 848–850).

There is currently no method for deciding which smoker should receive bupropion or nicotine replacement therapy (NRT) (*Br J Cardiol* 2005; **12**: 37). However, NRT is regarded as the pharmacological treatment of choice in the management of smoking cessation.

What are the NICE recommendations for smoking cessation treatments?

In April 2002, NICE recommended the use of bupropion and NRT for smokers who wish to quit. The guidance states that NRT or bupropion should normally only be prescribed when smokers have made a commitment to stop smoking on or before a certain date ('target stop date'), in conjunction with advice and encouragement to help them quit.

First prescriptions of NRT or bupropion should only be enough to last until 2 weeks after the target stop date. Normally, this will be 2 weeks for NRT. For bupropion it will be 3–4 weeks, because bupropion should be taken for about 1 week before the target stop date. Smokers should only be given a second prescription for NRT or bupropion if they can show they are still trying to stop smoking.

The Department of Health have recently produced health improvement targets for England to aim to reduce adult smoking rates from 26% in 2002 to 21% or less by 2010. (Department of Health. *National Standards, Local Action: Health and Social Care Standards Planning Framework.* London: DOH, 2004.)

Other treatments

The effectiveness of other treatments – namely aversion therapy, acupuncture, hypnotherapy and exercise – is as yet uncertain.

What is the cycle of change and how can it be used for smoking cessation?

There are undoubtedly certain times when a patient will be more receptive to advice on stopping smoking. Smoking cessation should not be regarded as a dichotomous process (cessation or not), but rather as a continuum that entails several stages. DiClemente and Prochaska's cycle of readiness to change (see Figure below) has been used to describe the psychological processes involved in many patterns of human behaviour and lends itself very well to smoking cessation (*J Consult Clin Psychol* 1991; **59**: 295–304). It is important to know the 'cycle of change' as it can be applied to various aspects of clinical practice, and can be very useful to discuss in the viva examination!

Precontemplation

This is the stage at which the patient is happy at being a smoker and does not contemplate stopping. Although brief intervention at this stage may not persuade them to give up, it may help them question their habit and move them nearer to the next stage.

Contemplation

This is the stage at which the patient is dissatisfied with being a smoker and is thinking about giving up (70% of adult smokers are at this stage!). During this stage, it can be effective to make the idea of quitting relevant to the patient, for example a patient recently diagnosed with heart disease.

Preparation

This is the stage at which the smoker is making serious plans to stop. It is therefore important to be supportive; discussion about smoking cessation treatments is most beneficial at this stage.

Action

This is the stage when maximum support should be given, as it is at this stage when the attempt to stop smoking is made.

Maintenance

This is the stage at which the patient tries to prevent relapse. This is often the most difficult time as enthusiasm often wears off quicker than withdrawal symptoms.

Relapse

This is obviously when the patient's attempt to stop smoking has been unsuccessful. This can either mean permanently giving up the idea of quitting smoking or thinking about it again in the future, whereby the patient would then re-enter the cycle at the precontemplation stage once more.

If the doctor or healthcare professional is unaware of where their patient is in this cycle of change, then any time and effort given regarding smoking cessation may be wasted.

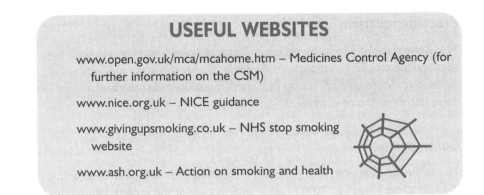

USEFUL WEBSITES

www.open.gov.uk/mca/mcahome.htm – Medicines Control Agency (for further information on the CSM)

www.nice.org.uk – NICE guidance

www.givingupsmoking.co.uk – NHS stop smoking website

www.ash.org.uk – Action on smoking and health

DiClemente and Prochaska's cycle of change

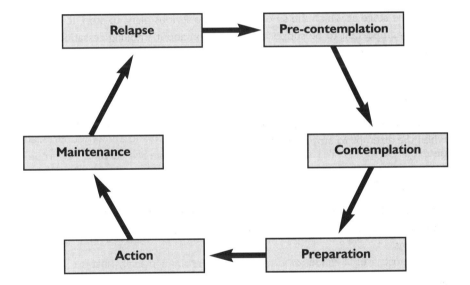

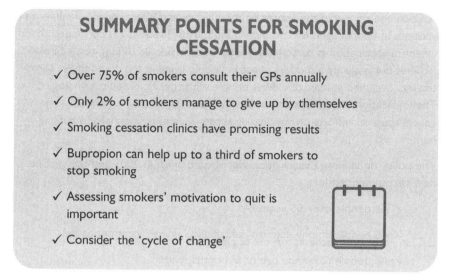

SUMMARY POINTS FOR SMOKING CESSATION

✓ Over 75% of smokers consult their GPs annually

✓ Only 2% of smokers manage to give up by themselves

✓ Smoking cessation clinics have promising results

✓ Bupropion can help up to a third of smokers to stop smoking

✓ Assessing smokers' motivation to quit is important

✓ Consider the 'cycle of change'

Influenza

During the winter months there is often an outbreak of influenza, caused by A or B virus, which results in a huge increased workload for both primary care teams and hospitals. Even when the incidence is low, it has been estimated that 3000–4000 deaths in the UK each year are from influenza-related causes. These deaths occur mainly in older people, but young children and immunosuppressed people are also at increased risk. Experts tell us that we are currently 'overdue' for a major flu pandemic and there has been much coverage in the media recently about bird flu.

Why do people require annual immunisation?

Unlike most viruses, influenza viruses A and B are antigenically unstable, and constantly alter their antigenic structure. Every year, the WHO makes recommendations about which strains should be included in the vaccine. The vaccine is an inactivated one and does not lead to influenza symptoms. The only contraindication is egg or chicken allergy.

What are the benefits of the influenza vaccine?

Overall, it is thought that influenza immunisation provides up to 70–80% protection against strains included in the vaccine, and helps prevent pneumonia, hospital admission and death (*N Engl J Med* 2000; **343**:1778–1787).

A Cochrane review in the *Lancet* on the efficacy and effectiveness of influenza vaccines in people aged 65 and older (2005; **366**: 1165–1174) concluded that influenza vaccination is reasonably effective for residents of long-term care facilities but has only a modest effect in people living in the community. The triallists excluded studies of elderly people with specific chronic pathologies. The implications of this systematic review seem to be that we should concentrate our efforts on vaccinating those living in residential and nursing homes.

The policy on influenza vaccination was altered again in 2005 and the vaccine is now recommended for:

✓ All people over 65 years old

✓ All people in long-stay residential and nursing accommodation

✓ All people (over the age of 6 months) with:

- Chronic respiratory disease, including asthma

- Chronic heart disease

- Chronic renal disease

- Diabetes mellitus

- Immunosuppression due to disease or treatment

- Chronic liver disease

- Carers of elderly or disabled patients, whose welfare might be compromised if the carer falls ill.

The GMS Contract categorises the provision of influenza immunisation as a directed enhanced service. Points are also awarded through the quality and outcomes framework (QOF) for immunising high-risk patients. Throughout the UK, the target for immunising those aged 65 and over is 70%. However, the QOF targets set for patients with COPD, diabetes, cerebrovascular disease and CHD are higher, at 85%.

What are the treatments for influenza?

Although vaccination remains the most important measure for reducing the burden of influenza, the viral neuraminidase inhibitors, zanamivir (Relenza®) and oseltamivir (Tamiflu®), are additional tools for treatment and prevention of influenza. Tamiflu® is currently thought to be the most effective treatment available should there be an outbreak of bird flu. Both drugs reduce replication of influenza viruses A and B. Amantadine is an older anti-viral drug and is no longer recommended for treatment of influenza. Worldwide resistance to these drugs has increased by 12% since the mid 1990s and some Asian countries have drug resistance frequencies exceeding 70% (*Lancet* 2005; **366**: 1175–1181).

Neuraminidase inhibitors have been shown to be clinically effective for the treatment of influenza in otherwise healthy adults and children as well as for the prevention of the disease (*BMJ* 2003; **326**: 1235–1240). When taken as prophylaxis they can decrease the likelihood of developing influenza by 70–90%. This systematic review showed that treating otherwise healthy adults and children with zanamivir and oseltamivir reduces the duration of symptoms by between 0.4 and 1.0 days. The treatment also lowers the risk of complications by 29–34% when it is given within 48 h of the onset of symptoms. However, there is still a lack of data on their efficacy in preventing serious influenza-related complications and mortality in groups at high risk – the elderly and people with co-morbidity.

Community studies have shown that seasonal prophylactic use of neuraminidase inhibitors administered after exposure in households and residential care would be clinically effective (*Vaccine* 2002; **20**: 2562–2578). There have been no studies to compare the response to treatment in vaccinated versus non-vaccinated people.

Oseltamivir, like zanamivir, is a neuraminidase inhibitor but unlike zanamivir it is readily absorbed from the gut so is an oral medication. In one study, 548 elderly people in residential homes were randomised to receive either oseltamivir or placebo for 6 weeks, starting when influenza was confirmed in the home or nearby (*J Am Geriatr Soc* 2001; **49**: 1025–1031). Oseltamivir was found to reduce the incidence of influenza from 4.4% with placebo to 0.4%. It seems to offer protection from influenza over and above that offered by the vaccination. It may be worthwhile, therefore, offering prophylaxis with oseltamivir to residents and staff in the event of an outbreak in a residential or nursing home (*Drug Ther Bull* 2002; **40**: 89–91).

When should zanamivir and oseltamivir be prescribed?

 NICE 2003 guidance

Flu is considered to be circulating in the community when consultations for flu rise to above 50 a week per 100,000 population, as monitored by the Royal College of General Practitioners' weekly returns monitoring service. The Public Health Laboratory Service must also have identified the circulation of a flu virus.

When influenza A or B is circulating in the community, the following guidance applies:

✓ Oseltamivir is recommended for post-exposure prophylaxis in at-risk adults and adolescents over the age of 13 who are not effectively protected by the influenza vaccine and who can commence the drug within 48 h of close contact with someone who has flu-like symptoms; prophylaxis is also recommended for residents in care establishments (regardless of influenza vaccination) who can commence oseltamivir within 48 h if influenza-like illness is present in the establishment.

✓ Oseltamivir and zanamivir are recommended to treat at-risk adults and children who can start treatment within 48 h of the onset of symptoms.

✓ Oseltamivir and zanamivir are NOT recommended for post-exposure prophylaxis or treatment of otherwise healthy individuals with influenza.

For the purposes of the guidance, 'high-risk' patients are defined as those with one or more of the following conditions: COPD, asthma, significant CVD (excluding hypertension), diabetes, chronic renal disease, immunosuppression and those over the age of 65.

Routine use of oseltamivir in the presence of influenza-like illness is not likely to be cost effective (*BMJ* 2004; **329**: 663).

It has been estimated that only 30% of self-diagnosed flu is actually due to influenza, and as there is no cheap, effective diagnostic test available, many people may be unnecessarily prescribed oseltamivir or zanamivir.

Why is there opposition to prescribing the neuraminidase inhibitors?

✓ The evidence to support them is still from small studies and many of the trials did not specifically recruit high-risk patients. The drug company's own product characteristics statement said that it had been unable to determine that zanamivir was effective in elderly patients and those with chronic conditions such as asthma and diabetes. In addition, there has been no published trial comparing its effect on influenza symptoms with symptomatic therapy (eg ibuprofen and paracetamol).

✓ There have been reports of fatal adverse reactions in patients with COPD and asthma in the USA. It has therefore been recommended that if zanamivir is to be prescribed for patients with airways disease, it should only be done under careful supervision with short-acting bronchodilators available.

✓ NICE originally refused to endorse the drug in 2000 and the *British Medical Journal* has criticised its U-turn as being a direct response to 'political clout'.

✓ The *Drug and Therapeutics Bulletin* will continue not to recommend zanamivir as part of the treatment of influenza as it is 'unconvinced of the benefits'. Certainly, the complications zanamivir reduces are minor – eg sinusitis. There is no evidence in benefit for major complications such as hospitalisation and death.

Finally, one study has found that most elderly people cannot actually use the zanamivir inhaler device correctly (*BMJ* 2001; **322**: 577–579). One of the authors of the study has advised that GPs need to spend at least 15 minutes teaching their elderly patients how to use the device; this is not realistic.

The possible emergence of resistance further limits the routine use of neuraminidase inhibitors (*Lancet* 2004; **364**: 759). National prescribing data show little inappropriate prescribing of zanamivir in the absence of high levels of influenza; prescriptions remained very low, at 499 in 2001, 190 in 2002, and 124 in 2003 (*BMJ* 2004; **329**: 999).

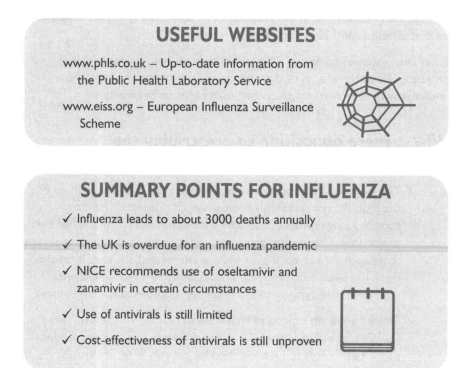

USEFUL WEBSITES

www.phls.co.uk – Up-to-date information from the Public Health Laboratory Service

www.eiss.org – European Influenza Surveillance Scheme

SUMMARY POINTS FOR INFLUENZA

✓ Influenza leads to about 3000 deaths annually

✓ The UK is overdue for an influenza pandemic

✓ NICE recommends use of oseltamivir and zanamivir in certain circumstances

✓ Use of antivirals is still limited

✓ Cost-effectiveness of antivirals is still unproven

CHAPTER 4:
PSYCHIATRY

CHAPTER 4:
PSYCHIATRY

Mental health National Service Framework

✓ Sets national standards for mental health services.

✓ Based on clinical evidence and sets out best practice for promoting mental health and treating mental illness.

✓ Accompanied by £700m for mental health services.

✓ Aims to iron out unacceptable variations around the country.

✓ Proposes further integration of health and social services.

Standards of care

1. Combat discrimination against individuals and groups with mental health problems, and promote their social inclusion.

2. Any service user who contacts their primary healthcare team with a common mental health problem should:

    • have their mental health needs identified and assessed

    • be offered effective treatments, including referral to specialist services if they require it.

3. Any individual with a common mental health problem should:

    • be able to make contact 24 h a day with local services

    • be able to use NHS Direct, as it develops, for first-level advice and referral on to specialist helplines or to local services.

4. All mental health service users should have a Care Programme Approach (CPA) and have a copy of a written care plan.

5. Each service user who is assessed as requiring a period of care away from their home should have timely access to an appropriate bed or place.

6. All individuals who provide regular and substantial care for a person on CPA should:

   - have an assessment of their caring, physical and mental health needs, repeated on at least an annual basis

   - have their own written care plan, which is given to them and implemented in discussion with them.

7. Prevent suicide. Reduce the suicide rate by at least one-fifth by 2010.

Criticisms

For many, the National Service Framework (NSF) arrived far too late. After years of chronic underfunding the expectation of achieving far-fetched idealistic targets within a short period seems unattainable.

Much of the document could easily be a party political broadcast on mental health. Should politics play such a large role?

Can NHS Direct really provide appropriate 24-h access?

GMS Contract and mental health

Mental health is also included in the new GP contract. In order to achieve maximum quality and outcomes framework (QOF) points, practices must achieve the following standards:

   - ✓ There must be a register of people with 'severe long-term mental health problems' in place.

   - ✓ 90% of patients with severe long-term mental health problems should have been reviewed in the previous 15 months.

   - ✓ 90% of patients on lithium therapy should have had their lithium levels checked in the previous 6 months.

   - ✓ 90% of patients receiving lithium should have a record of their serum creatinine and thyroid-stimulating hormone (TSH) in the previous 15 months.

   - ✓ 70% of patients on lithium should have lithium levels in the therapeutic range recorded within the previous 15 months.

Reforming the Mental Health Act, 2004

The Government published a new Draft Mental Health Bill for England and Wales on 8 September 2004.

Reforms were considered to be necessary for the following reasons

✓ The current 1983 Mental Health Act is largely based on a review of mental health legislation which took place in the 1950s; outmoded laws have failed to protect the public, patients or staff.

✓ Under existing mental health laws, the powers for compulsory treatment are for patients in hospital only, whilst the majority of patients today are treated in the community.

✓ Severely ill patients have been allowed to drift out of contact with mental health services and have been able to refuse treatment.

✓ Existing legislation has failed to provide adequate public protection from those whose risk to others arises from a severe personality disorder.

New proposals

✓ Community treatment orders, whereby compulsory treatment for psychiatric disease can be administered in the community as well as in hospital for certain patients.

✓ New independent body – the Mental Health Tribunal – to determine all longer-term use of compulsory powers, eg whether a patient should be forcibly treated in the community or detained in hospital.

✓ New right to independent advocacy.

✓ New safeguards for people with long-term mental incapacity.

✓ New Commission for Mental Health.

✓ Statutory requirement to develop care plans.

Implications for GPs

In Scotland

GPs are more likely to be called to give evidence at Mental Health Tribunals than under the old system.

GPs who give a second opinion for a continuing treatment order may be required to attend tribunals.

In England and Wales

✓ Community treatment orders may increase GPs' workload.

✓ GPs may need to be involved in Mental Health Tribunals, for patients treated in the community.

✓ GP practices may be designated as places where compulsory treatment is administered.

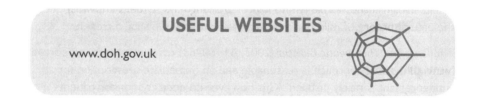

USEFUL WEBSITES

www.doh.gov.uk

Depression

Depression is a common condition, accounting for 12% of the total burden of non-fatal global disease. Prescribing of antidepressants has increased greatly in England in recent years.

Researchers estimate that by 2020 depression will be second only to ischaemic heart disease as the leading cause of disability-adjusted life years. Depression is common in general practice, with estimates ranging from 5.5% to 65% depending on the definition. It is thought that adult depression in England cost the country £9 billion in the year 2000, largely due to work incapacity (*Br J Psychiatry* 2003; **183**: 514–519).

The suicide rate in depressed people is at least eight times higher than that of the general population. Most people who complete suicide have a mental disorder, and in 50% of cases depression is associated with the suicide.

Depending on how depression is defined, GPs tend to miss between 50% and 75% of cases. Nine out of ten depressed patients are treated only in primary care and up to two-thirds of suicide victims contact a GP in the four weeks before the death. Like hypertension, depression is subject to a rule of halves – only half of depressed patients seek help from doctors, half are detected in primary care, half receive treatment with only half completing it: fewer than 10% finish a therapeutic course of treatment.

As GPs, we see distressed, tearful people every day and can sometimes wrongly label them as being depressed. Conversely, many of the patients whom we regularly treat for chronic, physical diseases (for example chronic obstructive pulmonary disease (COPD) and stroke) have underlying depression, which we fail to diagnose. This is important, as treating psychological distress can ameliorate physical disease; for example, treating depression in the elderly may improve pain scores (*JAMA* 2003; **290**: 2428).

Mild depression

As GPs, we see more cases of mild depression than major depression. This may be nothing more than a self-limiting reaction to adverse life events, but still results in significant morbidity and loss of working days. Little is known about the natural history of mild depression and about how we should treat it.

The *Drug and Therapeutic Bulletin* (2003; **41**: 60–63) concludes that a supportive 'watchful waiting approach is reasonable and an immediate prescription for an antidepressant is rarely justified'. GPs however do need to monitor patients with mild depression, in order to pick up those who develop a chronic problem. NICE concurs that there is little evidence to support the use of antidepressants in mild depression (see guidance below).

NICE guidelines 'Management of depression in primary and secondary care' December 2004

Key points

1. Screening should be undertaken in primary care and general hospital settings for depression in high-risk patients, eg those with a past history of depression, significant physical disability or dementia.

Screening can take place using two questions:

During the past month, have you often been bothered by feeling down, depressed or hopeless?

During the last month, have you often been bothered by having little interest or pleasure in doing things?

A positive response rate to both questions was found to have a 97% sensitivity and 67% specificity rate (*BMJ* 2003; **327**: 1144)

2. Antidepressants are not recommended in mild depression; if the patient is willing, it is reasonable to use a 'watchful waiting' strategy and to arrange review within two weeks. All patients with mild depression should be encouraged to follow a structured and supervised exercise programme, in which they participate in a 45- to 60-minute exercise session up to three times a week for 10–12 weeks.

3. Health care professionals should consider recommending a guided self-help programme based on cognitive behavioural therapy (CBT) for patients with mild depression.

4. Psychological treatment comprising six to eight sessions over 10–12 weeks should be considered for patients with mild or moderate depression. This treatment should be specifically focused on depression and might consist of CBT, counselling or problem-solving therapy.

5. When the decision has been made to initiate antidepressant medication in primary care, a selective serotonin-reuptake inhibitor (SSRI) should be used initially. This is because SSRIs are as effective as tricyclics but are less likely to be discontinued due to side-effects (*BMJ* 2003; **326**: 1014–1017).

6. For patients with severe depression, a combination of antidepressants and individual CBT should be offered.

7. Patients should be warned about discontinuation symptoms that might occur on abruptly stopping therapy. Treatment should generally be tailed off slowly over the course of 4 weeks. Venlafaxine is more likely to produce discontinuation symptoms than other drugs and should only be initiated by a specialist or by a GP with a special interest in psychiatry.

8. Patients who have had two or more depressive episodes in the recent past should be advised to continue antidepressants for two years.

Should we screen for depression?

The advice on screening for depression is still controversial. A recent Cochrane review of 12 studies (including 5693 patients) concluded that screening for depression had little, if any, effect on detection and management of depression or on patient outcomes (*Cochrane Library* 2005, issue 4). There was no evidence found that screening at-risk groups is beneficial.

An interesting editorial discusses the pros and cons of screening, arguing that since depression does not have a 'pre-clinical' phase, screening is hardly justified and does not fulfil Wilson's criteria (see Chapter 8, Cancer) (*Br J Gen Pract* 2005; **55**: 659–660). The author proposes that NICE is referring to 'case-finding' rather than screening and that diagnosis of any mental health disorder may require more than one consultation.

NICE recommends that we use guided self-help CBT programmes for people with mild depression. However, many GPs do not yet have access to such programmes. This will change in the future, as Primary Care Trusts (PCTs) become obliged to provide us with these resources. One study has recently shown that self-help CBT can be successfully delivered over the internet for patients with mild to moderate depression (*Br J Psychiatry* 2005; **187**: 456–461).

1. Effectiveness of SSRIs and low dose TCAs in treating depression in primary care (*Am J Med* 2005; **118**: 1087–1093)

✓ Meta-analysis involving 15 trials based in primary care, most only short-term.

✓ Relative rate of improvement was 1.37 for SSRIs and 1.26 for tricyclic antidepressants (TCAs).

This seems to contradict the findings of a recent Cochrane review (*Cochrane Library* 2005, issue 4) that examined trials comparing antidepressants with 'active' placebos, (ie placebos containing active substances which mimic the side-effects of antidepressants). Only small differences were found in favour of antidepressants in terms of improvements in mood. The authors concluded that the beneficial effects of antidepressants may be generally overestimated and their placebo effects may be underestimated.

2. Antidepressant drugs and generic counselling for treatment of major depression in primary care (*BMJ* 2001; **322**: 772–775)

The objective of this study was to compare the efficacy of antidepressant drugs and generic counselling for treating mild to moderate depression in general practice.

✓ RCT with patient-preference arms followed up at 8 weeks and 12 months.

✓ Generic counselling was found to be as effective as antidepressants for mild to moderate depressive illness.

✓ Patients receiving antidepressants recovered more quickly.

✓ 12 months after starting treatment generic counselling was as effective as antidepressants.

✓ Patients who chose counselling may benefit more than those with no strong preference.

However, this was a small study and used non-standardised counselling by experienced professionals.

3. General practice based intervention to prevent repeat episodes of deliberate self-harm: cluster randomised controlled trial (*BMJ* 2002; **324**: 1254–1257)

This large English study looked at whether a GP-based intervention on self-harm can reduce its incidence. We already know that:

1. Deliberate self-harm (DSH) is a serious clinical problem in England and Wales, accounting for an estimated 140,000 hospital presentations each year.

2. Some two-thirds of suicide victims contact a GP in the month before they kill themselves.

3. 15–23% of patients will be seen for treatment of a subsequent episode of deliberate self-harm within one year.

4. 3–5% of those who harm themselves die by suicide within 5–10 years.

   ✓ This was an RCT involving 98 practices who were assigned in equal numbers to an intervention or a control group.

   ✓ The intervention consisted of a letter from the GP inviting the patient to consult, and guidelines on the assessment and management of deliberate self-harm for the GP to use in consultations. Control patients received usual GP care.

   ✓ 1932 patients participated. The patients were registered with the study practices and had attended accident and emergency departments at one of four local district general hospitals in the Bath and Bristol area after an episode of deliberate self-harm.

✓ The primary outcome was a repeat episode of deliberate self-harm in the 12 months after the index episode. The study also looked at the number of repeat episodes and time to first repeat.

✓ The results showed that the incidence of repeat episodes of deliberate self-harm was not significantly different for patients in the intervention group compared with the control group.

✓ The treatment seemed to be beneficial for people with a history of deliberate self-harm, but it was associated with an adverse effect in people for whom the index episode was their first episode.

✓ The most effective management for patients who self-harm is not yet clear. One study has suggested that CBT might help to reduce the frequency of suicide attempts in patients with a history of deliberate self-harm; patients treated with CBT were 50% less likely to attempt suicide again in 18 months of follow-up, although interestingly, suicidal ideation was similar in both groups (*JAMA* 2005; **294**: 563–570).

SSRIs and suicide rates; Committee on the Safety of Medicines (CSM) review

Public confidence in the ability of GPs to manage depression has been knocked by current concerns about SSRIs, exaggerated in the media. Guidelines and advice have been produced by the Medicines and Healthcare Products Regulatory Agency (MHRA) concerning the prescription of antidepressants. The committee's advice, which has been incorporated into information for prescribers and patients, concerns withdrawal reactions, dose changes and suicidal behaviour.

✓ The CSM safety review concluded that the balance of risks and benefits of SSRIs in adults remains positive.

✓ There is thought to be no advantage in increasing the dose above the standard recommended daily dosage, and patients should be maintained on the lowest effective dose of their medication.

✓ Regular review is important.

✓ There was found to be no clear evidence of increased risk of self-harm or suicidal thoughts in adults aged over 18 although such an effect could not be ruled out. There was found to be insufficient evidence from clinical trial data to conclude that there is any marked difference between different SSRIs, or between SSRIs and other antidepressants, with respect to their influence on suicidal behaviour.

One meta-analysis reviewed 477 published and unpublished placebo-controlled SSRI studies, involving over 40,000 participants (*BMJ* 2005; **330**: 385). The researchers found no increased risk for completed suicides with SSRIs overall but did find modest, nearly significant evidence of an association between SSRI use and an increase in deliberate self-harm. They estimated that one such event would occur for every 759 patients treated.

A systematic review of 345 trials (with 36,000 subjects) found that SSRI use was associated with an increased risk of suicide attempts compared to placebo, but not compared with tricyclics (*BMJ* 2005; **330**: 396). The risk for completed suicide did not increase with the use of SSRIs compared to placebo. There were only 24 completed suicides reported overall.

It is worth noting that suicide rates have been declining steadily over the past 15 years in the USA, while prescriptions for SSRIs have increased exponentially. It is generally accepted that SSRIs are associated with a reduction (rather than an increase) in suicide rate in adults. The association in children is less clear. In adolescents, SSRIs other than fluoxetine have shown limited benefit and may increase the risk of suicide.

Antidepressant use in children and adolescents

Major depressive disorder is thought to have a point prevalence of about 1–2% in school-age children and 2–5% in adolescents. NICE guidelines recommend that antidepressants should only be initiated by a specialist for patients under 18. Psychological treatments should always be tried first.

There is no antidepressant in the UK that currently has a Marketing Authorisation for young people under 18 years old. Despite this, the CSM concluded that it is reasonable to prescribe fluoxetine for this age group if it is clinically indicated. The CSM has advised that only specialists should prescribe other antidepressants.

SSRIs and gastrointestinal bleeding

There was a review of this subject in a recent *Drug and Therapeutics Bulletin* (2004; **41**(3)). The estimated absolute risk increase of gastrointestinal (GI) bleeding is thought to be 3 extra episodes per 1000 patients treated; similar to the extra risk experienced by users of non-steroidal anti-inflammatory drugs (NSAIDs) or aspirin. The risk is higher in the elderly and in those being treated with concomitant aspirin or NSAIDs. Fluoxetine, sertraline and paroxetine are more likely to cause a bleed than other drugs in this group, but there is a relative risk of abnormal bleeding of 1.9 even with the other SSRIs (*Arch Intern Med* 2004; **164**: 2367–2370).

Post-natal depression

✓ This is a common problem, affecting about 70,000 women/year in the UK (approximately 13% of deliveries).

✓ Many recover spontaneously.

✓ 50% are still depressed at 6 months.

✓ One-third go on to develop a chronic, recurrent mood disorder.

✓ It is associated with disturbances in the mother–infant relationship, which in turn has an adverse impact on child cognitive and emotional development.

✓ Depression is more likely if there is previous psychiatric history, social problems or bereavement; this should be assessed antenatally.

✓ The Edinburgh Post-natal Depression Score is a validated detection tool.

Post-natal depression can have profound short- and long-term effects on maternal morbidity, the new infant and the family as a whole. A recent Cochrane review concluded that it is not known whether antidepressants are an effective and safe choice for treatment of this disorder (*Cochrane Library* 2005, issue 4). The authors could only identify one small randomised controlled trial which looked at fluoxetine and CBT in the treatment of post-natal depression. It was not possible to draw conclusions from this. More trials are needed to investigate the effectiveness of antidepressants and their place in treatment of post-natal depression, particularly in breastfeeding women.

Post-traumatic stress disorder (PTSD)

Typical symptoms include:

✓ Re-experiencing (eg flashbacks, nightmares, repetitive, intrusive images).

✓ Avoidance; avoiding people, situations or circumstances that are associated with the traumatic event.

✓ Hyperarousal; hypervigilance for threat, insomnia, exaggerated startle response.

✓ Emotional numbing with a sense of detachment from others and difficulty in experiencing feelings. This may be associated with amnesia for part of the event.

✓ Depression.

✓ Drug or alcohol misuse.

✓ Anger.

✓ Somatisation, with inexplicable physical symptoms.

Although symptoms usually develop immediately after the traumatic event, their onset may be delayed in a minority of patients (<15%).

NICE guidelines March 2005; key points

✓ Debriefing should NOT be offered routinely to people who have experienced a traumatic event.

✓ Watchful waiting is recommended in mild cases of PTSD where symptoms are mild.

✓ Patients with severe symptoms or with severe PTSD in the first month after the traumatic event should be offered trauma-focused CBT.

✓ All people with PTSD should be offered a course of trauma-focused psychological treatment.

✓ Treatment may be effective even when problems present many years after the traumatic event.

✓ Drug treatments should not be used as a first-line treatment in preference to trauma-focused CBT, but may be an option for adults who decline psychological treatment; in particular mirtazapine and paroxetine.

✓ Consider screening people at high risk of developing PTSD one month after the traumatic event.

PTSD editorial (*Br J Gen Pract* 2004; **54**: 83–85)

This points out that the definition of a traumatic stressful event has been broadened to include learning about an actual or threatened event suffered by another, eg the unexpected death of a friend or being the parent of a child diagnosed with a serious illness. Furthermore, the traumatic stressor no longer has to be a major life-threatening event, so may include incidents of bullying at school or at work.

Other important points:

- ✓ Prevalence in the UK is unclear.

- ✓ A 1995 survey in the USA indicated a 7.8% lifetime prevalence in those aged 15–55 years.

- ✓ People with PTSD are frequent users of health care.

- ✓ They can present with multiple somatic symptoms.

- ✓ There are high levels of co-morbidity with other mental conditions (eg anxiety, depression and substance misuse).

- ✓ Consequently, it is likely that PTSD is significantly under-diagnosed in the general population.

- ✓ In conclusion there should be a heightened awareness among GPs of this condition.

Schizophrenia

There is thought to be a 0.2–1% lifetime prevalence in the general population. It is among the leading causes of disability worldwide.

It is estimated to cost England and Wales £1 billion per year (about 3% of total NHS expenditure).

- ✓ There is growing evidence that the early stages of schizophrenia are critical in forming and predicting the course and outcome of the disorder. Rapid diagnosis and early referral are therefore very important, as is initiating treatment early.

- ✓ Unfortunately, schizophrenia typically remains undetected for 2–3 years; probably due to its often insidious onset. Also, there may be reluctance in making this potentially stigmatising diagnosis. Diagnosis is often made later in socially deprived groups (*BMJ* 2001; **323**: 1398).

- ✓ The aim of primary treatment is rapid remission, and strategies that result in a minimum of side-effects should be used.

NICE guidance

Guidelines on core interventions for the treatment and management of people with schizophrenia in primary and secondary care were published in December

2002. The recommendations were made after a review of over 200 trials. In March 2003, the National Collaborating Centre for Mental Health (NCCMH), which is funded by NICE, launched an interactive training package for healthcare professionals to help them to become familiar with NICE guidance (accessible by the Royal College of Psychiatrists website and takes about 1 h to work through: www.rcpsych.ac.uk/cru/sts/index.htm).

The aim of the NICE guidance is to improve the experience and outcomes of care for people with schizophrenia (referred to as 'service users'). Summary points are listed:

✓ The importance of obtaining informed consent before initiation of treatment wherever possible is stressed.

✓ The development of advance directives regarding the choice of treatment is recommended.

✓ All newly diagnosed or suspected cases should be urgently referred to secondary care.

✓ GPs should consider starting atypical antipsychotic drugs if there are acute symptoms.

✓ The following oral atypical antipsychotic drugs are recommended for first-line treatment in newly diagnosed schizophrenia because of the lower risk of extrapyramidal symptoms – amisulpride, olanzapine, quetiapine, risperidone and zotepine.

✓ Psychological treatments especially CBT and family therapy should be available as treatment options.

✓ The physical health of people with schizophrenia is best monitored in primary care.

✓ Practice case registers are recommended (now a GMS quality indicator).

✓ The following points should be covered in the annual review and recorded in the notes:

1. Cardiovascular disease (CVD) risk factors (including obesity and smoking).

2. Side-effects of treatment, including extrapyramidal side-effects.

3. Consider the risk of diabetes.

4. Consider hyperprolactinaemia.

The yearly cost of maintenance on older style antipsychotics is £70, whereas for atypical drugs it averages £1220. NICE estimates that the cost to the NHS of making these drugs freely available will be £70 million a year, but that this will be offset by an expected shift away from inpatient care to cheaper community-based care.

All patients should have a care plan and GPs should function in multidisciplinary teams.

Side-effects of atypical antipsychotic drugs

This subject was reviewed in the *Drug and Therapeutic Bulletin* (August 2004; **42** (8)). It concluded that there is an urgent need for more clinical trials to clarify the differences between the drugs available currently.

Most side-effects are dose related so the advice is to start at a low dose and increase slowly.

- ✓ **EPS**: the incidence is generally low but can occur at the upper end of the licensed dose range with amisulpride, olanzapine and risperidone.

- ✓ **Hyperprolactinaemia**: there is no correlation between drug dose, prolactin concentration and occurrence of symptoms. Long-term and potentially harmful effects of sustained hyperprolactinaemia and secondary suppression of gonadotrophins is not known (eg on bone density and fertility). Quetiapine and olanzapine are 'prolactin-sparing'.

- ✓ **Weight gain**: this is clearly an important CVD and diabetes risk factor and occurs most commonly with clozapine and olanzapine. Body mass index (BMI) should be measured before starting treatment and at regular intervals thereafter.

- ✓ **Diabetes mellitus**: the prevalence in patients with schizophrenia is twice that of the general population. Antipsychotics may increase this risk further – it is not clear if this excess risk is solely due to the weight gain associated with their use. The risk is thought to be highest with olanzapine and clozapine.

- ✓ **Dyslipidaemia**: studies suggest this is linked to weight gain. Olanzapine and clozapine tend to be associated with adverse changes in serum concentrations of triglyceride and cholesterol.

- ✓ **Stroke**: olanzapine and risperidone are associated with an increased risk of stroke in elderly patients when used in the management of dementia (see Chapter 5, The Elderly). Any antipsychotic should be avoided in elderly patients with risk factors for cerebrovascular events.

It is recommended that fasting glucose, lipids and blood pressure (BP) are checked before treatment is started, after 3 months and then again as appropriate

Atypical antipsychotics, patients value the lower incidence of extrapyramidal side-effects (*BMJ* 2000; **321**: 1360)

This editorial appeared in the *British Medical Journal* alongside a systematic review of atypicals. Points raised were:

- ✓ There was no clinically significant evidence of superiority in efficacy, or for that matter tolerability, for atypical antipsychotics as a group.

- ✓ Atypical antipsychotics account for nearly three out of four new prescriptions for antipsychotics in North America.

- ✓ Atypicals have a lower incidence of extrapyramidal side-effects.

- ✓ Extrapyramidal side-effects are not just incidental 'side' effects but the central factor in many patients' agendas.

- ✓ Extrapyramidal effects by themselves have been related to a poor outcome, a compromised compliance, secondary negative symptoms, cognitive parkinsonism and depression as well as the long-term risk of tardive dyskinesia.

- ✓ It may turn out that the real superiority of atypicals is not in their antipsychotic abilities but in their ability to control ancillary symptoms related to mood, cognition, hostility and a higher level of compliance.

- ✓ Atypical agents have their own new side-effects such as weight gain and diabetes.

Crisis resolution teams

The NHS plan and the Department of Health 'Mental Health Policy Implementation Guide' both stipulate that crisis resolution teams should manage acute psychiatric exacerbations suffered by patients with severe mental illness. The idea is to contain the crisis at an early stage and to prevent hospital admission.

A recent RCT set out to evaluate the effectiveness of one such crisis resolution team based in Islington in London (*BMJ* 2005; **331**: 599–602). Two hundred and sixty residents who were experiencing significant mental health crises (sufficient to be severe enough to consider hospital admission) were randomised to standard care from community mental health teams and inpatient services or to acute care, including a 24-h crisis resolution team. Patients in the latter group were less likely to be admitted to hospital in the 8 weeks after the crisis, though compulsory admission was not significantly reduced.

Other treatments

'Integrated therapy', consisting of assertive community treatment with programmes for family involvement and social skills training, may improve clinical outcome and adherence to treatment for patients who experience their first psychotic episode (*BMJ* 2005; **330**: 602–605). In this trial, integrated therapy was provided for 2 years.

Eating disorders

The NSF for mental health has outlined the need to improve the standard of health care for people with eating disorders. In January 2004, NICE issued guidance on core interventions in the management of anorexia nervosa, bulimia nervosa and related eating disorders. The following recommendations were made:

- ✓ A comprehensive assessment should take place, including physical, social and psychological needs.
- ✓ GPs should take responsibility for the initial assessment and co-ordination of care when a patient presents.
- ✓ Get help early; patients with eating disorders should be assessed and treated as soon as possible.
- ✓ Where laxative abuse is present, patients should be advised to gradually reduce laxative use and be informed that laxative use does not significantly reduce calorie absorption.
- ✓ The right to confidentiality of children and adolescents with eating disorders should be respected.

Screening in primary care

Target groups should include:

- ✓ Young women with low BMI.

✓ Non-overweight patients consulting with excessive weight concerns.

✓ Women with menstrual disturbances or amenorrhoea.

✓ Patients with GI symptoms.

✓ Those with physical signs of starvation or repeated vomiting.

✓ Children with poor growth.

Consider these simple screening questions:

Do you think you have an eating problem?

Do you worry excessively about your weight?

Anorexia nervosa

Most patients should be managed on an outpatient basis with psychological treatments (and physical monitoring). Therapies that may be effective include cognitive analytic therapy, cognitive behavioural therapy, interpersonal psychotherapy and family interventions. Psychological treatment should be for at least 6 months if done on an outpatient basis. Medication is not a primary treatment for anorexia nervosa. If an antidepressant is used, the doctor must remain vigilant for cardiac side-effects as compromised cardiovascular function.

Bulimia nervosa

Patients may be considered for an evidence-based self-help programme with encouragement and support from health professionals. There is good evidence for a specific form of CBT for bulimia which should normally be for 16–20 sessions. SSRI antidepressants (specifically fluoxetine) can reduce the frequency of binge eating and purging. Long-term effects are unknown.

How well are these guidelines being implemented?

In February 2005, the Eating Disorders Association produced a report that was highly critical of GPs. The report surveyed 1700 sufferers, carers and professionals and compared the treatment actually provided to that recommended by the NICE guidelines. The report claimed that 40% of GPs failed to meet guidelines on identification and urgent referral. It also highlighted the shortage of specialist psychiatric services, so even when GPs did quickly identify cases, facilities were not readily available.

Alcohol

It has been estimated that alcohol misuse is costing England £6.4 billion per year through lost productivity, in terms of absence from work, unemployment and premature death; in addition, the direct costs to the NHS are £1.7 billion per year, with 150,000 hospital admissions. On average, every GP in England sees 364 heavy drinkers per year and 1 in 25 adults in the UK is dependent on alcohol. Alcohol misuse has been cited as the second most common preventable cause of death in the country after smoking. One-third of patients with mental illness have substance misuse problems and alcohol dependence is associated with an 80-fold increase in male depression and suicide.

The quantities of alcohol consumed in the UK have been rising since the 1950s, and this is especially marked amongst young people, with 16- to 24-year-olds drinking most heavily.

The government's 'Alcohol Harm Reduction Strategy for England' was published in 2004 (www.strategy.gov.uk), in an attempt to address some of the problems resulting from alcohol misuse. Critics have complained that the new extended licensing hours will offset any benefit that this strategy might bring.

Recommended limits

The government's 'sensible drinking guidelines' suggest:

✓ a maximum intake of 2–3 units per day for women and 3–4 for men, with two alcohol-free days after heavy drinking; continued alcohol consumption at the upper level is not advised;

✓ that intake of up to 2 units a day can have a moderately protective effect against heart disease for men over 40 and for post-menopausal women; and

✓ that some groups, such as pregnant women and those engaging in potentially dangerous activities (such as operating heavy machinery), should drink less or nothing at all.

The recommended upper limits for alcohol consumption suggested by the Royal College of Physicians (RCP)/ Royal College of General Practitioners (RCGP)/ Royal College of Psychiatrists (RCPsych) are 14 units (1 unit being equivalent to 8–10 g of alcohol) per week for women and 21 for men. Around a quarter of the adult population drink in excess of these limits; 6.4 m drink up to 35 units a week (women) or 50 units a week (men). A further 1.8 m, two-thirds of them men, drink above even these levels.

We know from population studies that non-drinkers and heavy drinkers have higher all-cause mortality rates than light drinkers; this is known as the U-shaped curve. In systematic reviews of all-cause mortality, the risk has been shown to be lowest for men drinking 7–14 units a week and for women drinking under 7 units a week (*J Clin Epidemiol* 1999; **52**: 967–975).

The alcohol reduction strategy for England 2004

The four key aims of the strategy are listed below:

1. Improved and better targeted education and communication; to make people (especially the young) aware of sensible drinking guidelines and to change our culture of binge-drinking (how does this tie in with extended licensing hours?).

2. Better identification and treatment of alcohol problems; for example in general practice.

3. Better co-ordination and enforcement of the current framework to tackle crime and antisocial behaviour and support for victims of alcohol-related crime.

4. Encouraging the alcoholic drinks industry to promote more responsible drinking and take a role in reducing alcohol-related harms.

Criticisms of the government's alcohol reduction strategy

Many groups feel that the strategy just doesn't go far enough. The RCP made the following criticisms:

✓ There is undue dependence on voluntary action by the drinks industry.

✓ There is no clear plan with proper outcome targets for any partnership with the industry.

✓ There are calls for pilot schemes for brief interventions when the evidence from pilot studies is already available.

✓ There is undue emphasis on auditing existing alcohol treatment services rather than properly funding and extending them.

✓ The strengths, such as the emphasis on earlier detection and prevention of harm, are not backed up by funding.

✓ The opportunity to use the new GP contract to develop primary care targets has been missed.

✓ The opportunities to use presentations to A&E departments and acute hospital wards are not developed.

✓ There is no requirement for acute hospital trusts or PCTs to develop a coherent alcohol strategy and no targets to drive progress.

✓ Little or no attention is given to the measures that are of proven benefit in reducing harm – price and access. While the government fears electoral repercussions of such levers, it misses an opportunity to engage the population in proper and responsible debate.

Identifying problem drinkers

Currently, it is estimated that only one-third of problem drinkers are known to their GPs. Most GPs rely on the use of unstructured questions and blood tests, both of which are unreliable in detecting heavy drinkers. One study confirmed the poor reliability of blood tests and also compared five different alcohol screening questionnaires (*Br J Gen Practice* 2001; **51**: 206–217), showing that they all performed much better than blood tests, except for the CAGE questionnaire. The **Audit** questionnaire is 92% sensitive and 93% specific.

It is unclear whether routine screening for excessive alcohol intake could be done effectively in the primary care setting. A systematic review (*BMJ* 2003; **327**: 536–542) concluded that of 1000 patients screened using a health questionnaire, only 25 were eligible for brief intervention in the form of advice, information, or feedback. Of these 25, less than 3 reported that they had cut down their alcohol consumption to within recommended limits after a year.

Alcohol and the GMS Contract

Specialist treatment of alcohol misuse is a national enhanced service. Practices are required to keep an up to date register of patients who admit to misusing alcohol and are funded to provide services such as support of behavioural change and detoxification.

Does AA work?

Attending Alcoholics Anonymous may improve the chances of staying abstinent: a small study (*Alcohol Alcoholism* 2003; **38**: 421–426) demonstrated that after 6 months of attending AA meetings, participants drank significantly less alcohol, drank less often and reported fewer problems related to drink. They also had fewer psychological problems and enjoyed a better quality of life.

1. Cost-effectiveness of treatment for alcohol problems: findings of the randomised UK Alcohol Treatment Trial (UKATT) (UKATT Research Team, *BMJ* 2005; **331**: 544–543)

This trial set out to compare the cost-effectiveness of 'social behaviour and network therapy' with that of 'motivational enhancement therapy'. Both therapies have previously been shown to be effective in randomised controlled trials (*Alcoh Clin Exp Res* 1998; **22**: 1300–1311 and *BMJ* 2005; **331**: 541–544).

Social behaviour and network therapy aims to help clients build social networks to support change in their drinking and associated behaviours; participants received up to eight 50-minute sessions. Motivational enhancement therapy combines counselling in the motivational style with objective individual feedback from earlier assessment. Participants were given up to three 50-minute sessions.

- ✓ There were 742 clients included, all with alcohol problems; 617 (83.2%) were interviewed at 12 months and full economic data were obtained from 608.

- ✓ The main economic measures were quality-adjusted life-years (QALYs), cost of trial treatments and consequences for public sector resources (eg health care, social services and the criminal justice system).

- ✓ Both therapies saved about 5 times as much in expenditure on health, social and criminal justice services as they cost. Both therapies were similarly cost-effective.

- ✓ Trial participants reported highly significant reductions in drinking and associated problems and costs.

- ✓ The average cost of social behaviour and network therapy was £221 per patient, compared to £129 for motivational enhancement therapy.

2. Editorial: Dying for a drink (*BMJ* 2001; **323**: 817–818)

This focused on developing strategies to reduce suicide amongst those with alcohol-use disorders.

The following points were raised:

- ✓ There is a consistently high reported prevalence of alcohol-use disorders among people who commit suicide (eg 56% in New York, 43% in Northern Ireland).

- ✓ The lifetime risk of suicide is 7% in patients with alcohol dependence.

- ✓ In the Northern Ireland suicide study, the estimated risk of suicide in the presence of current alcohol misuse or dependence was eight times greater than in its absence.

- ✓ 89% of suicides with alcohol dependence in the Irish study had at least one other co-morbid mental disorder.

- ✓ The 5-year report of the National Confidential Inquiry into Suicide and Homicide by People with Mental Illness has revealed that 40% of people who commit suicide in England and Wales who have been in contact with mental health services within 1 year of death have a history of alcohol misuse (53% in Scotland) and 19% have misused both alcohol and drugs (26% in Scotland).

- ✓ Patients who attempt suicide should be assessed and treated for alcohol misuse.

USEFUL CONTACT INFORMATION

Alcohol Concern – national umbrella body for >500 local agencies tackling alcohol-related problems and providing support for families of alcoholics. It funds a helpline called the 'drink line' that can put patients in touch with a local agency that will provide help with detoxification and general support.

Helpline number 0800 9178282

www.alcoholconcern.org.uk

Alcoholics Anonymous

Helpline 020 78330022 or 0141 2262214 for Scotland

Drug misuse

Over 3 million people in the UK use illegal drugs every year, of whom 500,000 use drugs such as heroin and cocaine. One per cent of regular heroin users die each year, compared to 0.001% of cocaine users. The cost of harm to health and/or social functioning from heroin and/or crack use is estimated to be £5 billion per year.

GMS Contract and drug misuse

This is a national enhanced service. Practices are funded to develop practice guidelines on the management of drug users, to treat dependent users (with support, eg from shared care drug services), to ensure that co-existing physical, emotional, social and legal problems are addressed and to act as a resource for practice colleagues.

 Drug Misuse and Dependence – Guidelines on Clinical Management. Department of Health, 1999

This guideline, first published in 1991, was updated in 1999 in the light of recent advances. Great discrepancy exists throughout the UK in terms of provision of services. Many of the points in the plan caused a lot of controversy and still remain topical in the GP press. In summary from the guidelines:

- ✓ The total number of drug misusers presenting for treatment in the 6 months ending March 1998 was around 30,000.

- ✓ 54% of these users were in their twenties.

- ✓ 1 in 7 (15%) were aged under 20 years.

- ✓ The ratio of males to females was 3:1.

- ✓ 55% reported heroin as their main drug of misuse.

- ✓ Methadone was the next most frequently reported main drug of misuse at 13%, followed by cannabis and amphetamines, both at 9%.

- ✓ Self-reported drug use amongst those aged 16–59 years in England and Wales in 1996 showed that approximately 1 in 10 had used illegal drugs in the last year, and that 1 in 20 (6%) had done so in the last month.

- ✓ 60% of people arrested test positive for illegal drugs.

✓ People who are involved in drugs may have multiple social and medical problems.

✓ Doctors everywhere must expect to see drug misusers presenting for care and will need to be vigilant in looking for signs of drug misuse in their patients.

✓ It is the responsibility of all doctors to provide care for both general health needs and drug-related problems, whether or not the patient is ready to withdraw from drugs.

✓ This should include the provision of evidence-based interventions such as hepatitis B vaccination and hepatitis C screening.

✓ Medical practitioners should not prescribe in isolation, but should seek to liaise with other professionals who will be able to help with factors contributing to an individual's drug misuse.

✓ A multidisciplinary approach to treatment is therefore essential.

✓ Where there are no local specialist services with which a shared care agreement can be developed, it is the responsibility of the health authority to ensure that appropriate services are in place.

✓ There is good evidence for methadone maintenance treatment. Good initial assessment is important and there should be clear evidence of dependence, withdrawal and tolerance before treatment starts. Supervised consumption is recommended for the first 3 months and should be continued further if there are doubts about compliance.

✓ Prescribing is the doctor's responsibility and cannot be delegated. Clear records should be kept, and the doctor should regularly liaise with the dispensing pharmacist.

✓ No more than 1 weeks' supply should be given at any one time, except in exceptional circumstances.

✓ Regular clinical reviews are recommended, at least once every 3 months.

In 2002, the government updated its 1998 strategy 'Tackling drugs to build a better Britain'. Its original four aims remain the same:

1. To prevent young people from using drugs by prohibition and education.

2. To reduce the prevalence of drugs by tackling supply.

3. To reduce drug-related crime.

4. To reduce the demand for drugs by encouraging more problem users to accept treatment. The focus is on 'drugs that do the most harm' – namely heroin and crack cocaine.

Drugs used in opioid dependence substitution treatment

Methadone

Methadone maintenance treatment (MMT) has been shown to reduce illicit opioid use, reduce crime, decrease injecting activity and enhance social productivity (*BMJ* 1994; **309**: 997). There is a very real potential for toxicity however, and it is important to get the starting dose right, to avoid cumulative toxicity. After full assessment, oral liquid methadone should be started at 10–40 mg daily; particular care is needed above 30 mg as a starting dose, so if uncertainty exists, the starting dose should be 10–20 mg. The patient should then be stabilised over the next 6 weeks, probably so that they end up receiving between 60 and 120 mg daily. After stabilisation, dose reduction may be attempted, but only if the patient is willing to try; otherwise MMT can be continued indefinitely. The success rates of outpatient detoxification programmes are quite low, but a supportive home environment helps.

Buprenorphine

This is an opioid partial agonist/antagonist and comes in a sublingual preparation. It is now licensed for treatment of opioid dependence. It has less potential for overdose and has low euphoric effects at high doses. A Cochrane review (*Cochrane Library* issue 1, 2002) has examined the short-term management of opioid withdrawal with buprenorphine and concluded that although it seems to be effective, there is limited evidence at present.

Lofexidine

This is a non-opioid alpha agonist, which is licensed to relieve symptoms in patients undergoing detoxification. It has a similar action to clonidine, but causes less hypotension. It is only likely to be useful in patients whose average drug use is <1 g heroin per day (50 mg methadone equivalent) and with short drug histories.

Naltrexone

This is an opioid antagonist that should only be initiated in a drug addiction centre. It can only be used in highly motivated addicts who have remained drug free for 7–10 days. It is licensed as an 'adjunctive prophylactic therapy for maintenance of detoxified, formerly opioid-dependent patients'.

Should we be prescribing heroin?

In Holland, there has been some recent research looking at the safety and efficacy of supervised medical prescription of heroin to addicts not benefiting from methadone maintenance (*BMJ* 2003; **327**: 310–312). Five hundred and forty-nine heroin addicts were prescribed inhaled or injectable heroin over 12 months in two separate RCTs; heroin plus methadone was compared to methadone alone, in terms of physical and mental health and social functioning. Twelve months of treatment with heroin plus methadone was significantly more effective than treatment with methadone alone in both trials, whether given through injection or inhalation. The incidence of serious adverse events was similar across treatment conditions. The authors concluded that supervised co-prescription of heroin with methadone is feasible, and is more effective and probably as safe as methadone alone in reducing the many physical, mental and social problems of treatment-resistant heroin addicts.

A recent Home Office review has recommended an expansion of injectable heroin to patients within the NHS; however, it currently remains unclear which patients will benefit most from this type of treatment. A special Home Office license is required to allow doctors to prescribe heroin for the treatment of addiction. No such license is required for methadone. The main benefit of injection is probably harm reduction.

Cannabis

Cannabis was reclassified as a class C drug in early 2004.

Cannabis editorial (*Br J Gen Pract* 2003; **53**: 598–599)

In this editorial, Dr Gerada (project director of the RCGP Drug Training Programme) outlines the adverse effects of cannabis and makes the following key points:

✓ The reputation of cannabis as a safe drug can no longer be justified.

✓ Cannabis contains at least as many carcinogens as tobacco smoke.

✓ It is a markedly stronger drug than 20–30 years ago.

✓ It produces dependence in 5–10% of users.

✓ It impairs attention, memory and psychomotor performance.

✓ In large amounts, it can cause anxiety and depression and psychotic states.

✓ Three to four cannabis cigarettes a day can cause damage similar to smoking 20+ cigarettes per day.

✓ Robust evidence is required for the therapeutic benefits of cannabis (which must outweigh the risks).

Cannabis in Multiple Sclerosis study (CAMS) (*Lancet* 2003; 362: 1517–1526)

The aim of this large multicentre UK trial was to test the notion that cannabinoids have a beneficial effect on spasticity (primary outcome measure) and other symptoms related to multiple sclerosis (MS). It was an RCT including 630 patients with MS treated for 15 weeks with placebo or oral cannabis extract (delta–9-tetrahydrocannabinol, THC). Pain was assessed with a category rating scale and overall assessment took place at the end of the study.

✓ Treatment with cannabinoids **did not have a beneficial effect on spasticity** (this was assessed using the Ashworth scale which has been used in other studies and is thought to be the most reliable measure of spasticity but, as is outlined in the study discussion, spasticity is a complex symptom to objectively measure).

✓ There was a high placebo response (nearly 50% of those in the placebo group felt that their spasticity had improved).

✓ The group given cannabinoids reported an improvement in pain.

✓ There was also a beneficial effect on walking time (the median time taken to walk 10 m from baseline was reduced by 12% in those taking THC).

✓ The study concludes that there is some evidence that cannabinoids have a clinically useful role in MS but further research is needed using outcome measures that more adequately assess the effect of symptoms in chronic disease.

A cannabis-based drug called 'Sativex' is now available in Canada as a spray pump and is licensed for the relief of neuropathic pain.

Is cannabis safe?

There have been moves recently to decriminalise cannabis. People will no longer be automatically arrested for carrying 'small quantities for personal use only'. However, there are concerns about the safety of cannabis use, including a link between cannabis use in adolescence and an increased risk of psychosis in adulthood (*BMJ* 2002; **325**: 1212–1213). Early cannabis use (by the age of 15) confers a greater risk than does later use (by the age of 18), and this risk has been found to be specific to cannabis, as opposed to other recreational drugs, even after psychotic symptoms preceding the onset of cannabis use are controlled for. Cannabis use does not predict later depression.

BMA calls for Government action on drugs and driving (*BMJ* 2002; **324**: 632)

✓ The BMA has called on the UK Government to develop a campaign to highlight that taking drugs, whether prescribed, over the counter, or illegal, can impair driving capacity in a similar way to alcohol.

✓ The BMA has recommended that the Government should co-ordinate scientific research to establish effective drug-testing devices and should educate the public on the association between taking some drugs and impaired driving ability.

✓ To help publicise the problem, the BMA has developed a website that reviews trends in road traffic fatalities and injuries, as well as research on drugs and driving performance.

✓ The website highlights research from the Transport Research Laboratory warning that the number of people involved in fatal collisions who tested positive for illegal drugs increased sixfold between 1985–1987 and 1996–1999.

✓ The number of people testing positive for cannabis increased from 3% to 12%. Over the same period, the incidence of use of medicinal drugs and alcohol remained similar.

✓ Driving while unfit under the influence of drugs is an offence in the UK, and a driver faces the same penalties as for driving under the influence of alcohol.

✓ However, the law does not currently state any legal limits for drugs, as it does for alcohol, making it difficult to enforce legislation.

✓ The BMA is calling for this dilemma to be resolved by the development of appropriate testing devices.

✓ The BMA's initiative arose from a resolution passed at its annual meeting of representatives in 2001 to consider ways of supporting the police in their fight against drugs and driving.

Illegal drugs are found in 1 in 5 of those killed on the road. Doctors have a responsibility to report to the authorities any patients they know to be driving whilst taking drugs that might impair their consciousness.

USEFUL WEBSITES

www.bma.org.uk – This allows access to the BMA's drugs and driving website

USEFUL CONTACT INFORMATION

Council for Involuntary Tranquilizer Addiction; helpline for general public 0151 932 0102

National Drugs Helpline The National Drugs Helpline is a 24-h, 7-days a week, free and confidential telephone service that offers advice and information for those who are concerned, or have questions, about drugs. The service is available to anyone.

Helpline number 0800 776600

Parents Against Drug Abuse Helpline – 08457 023 867

Release (this is a legal advice helpline to support drug users, their family and friends and professionals) – tel 0845 4500 215

www.release.org.uk

Postgraduate Examination Resources

We subscribe to:

Medical Masterclass
www.medical-masterclass.com

Ask Library Staff for a personal account which gives you access and lets you store your history and progress. Covers MRCP Part 1 and 2, provides practice exams and allows you to choose specialty specific questions

Free resources:

MRCPass
www.mrcpass.com

Covering MRCP Part 1, offering 100+ free MCQ's and pass notes

Medexam.net
www.medexam.net

Register for free and get 2 days access to 1800+ 5-part questions for MRCP, MRCPGP, DipGerMed, PLAB

ReviseMRCP
www.revisemrcp.com

MedicineCPD
www.medicinecpd.co.uk

Free registration gives you access to best of 5 multiple choice MRCP questions

Exam Doctor
www.examdoctor.co.uk

A free 7 day trial gives you resources for: MRCP, MRCPCH, FRCR, MRCS Part 2/Part A:2, MRCOG, DRCOG, MRCGP, MRCPsych, FRCA, MCEM Part A, PLAB Part 1, FRCPath Haem Part 1: Paper 2

Exam Consult
www.examconsult.co.uk

50 free questions for Basic Science, Medical Finals and MRCP Part 2

Counselling

Q. What is counselling?

A. It is helping patients to identify, understand, come to terms with and cope with their problems.

Skills needed

Listening

Empathising

Reflecting

Clarifying

Summarising

Interpreting

Confronting

Motivating

Various counselling styles

- Directive — Counsellor acts prescriptively

- Informative — Counsellor provides information to help decision-making

- Confrontational — Counsellor challenges unhelpful thinking/behaviour

- Cathartic — Counsellor encourages expression of hidden thoughts/fears/guilt

- Catalytic — Counsellor encourages patient to establish own goal/take control

- Supportive — Counsellor provides acceptance, empathy, concern for patient's anxieties and needs

- Rogerian — Counsellor provides non-directive listening rather than advice, encouraging patient to make decisions based on own judgement

It has been known in the MRCGP exam to be asked for working examples of the above techniques, for example: 'Give an example of the use of catalytic intervention'.

Does it work?

Evidence suggests counselling in general practice is an effective therapy for psychosocial problems and minor affective disorders.

Some trials (not all) show that doctors:

- ✓ Identify more problems
- ✓ Prescribe fewer drugs
- ✓ Investigate less
- ✓ Refer less.

Patients:

- ✓ Get relief from symptoms
- ✓ Cope better with feelings
- ✓ Cope better with life
- ✓ Consult less often.

More information is needed on the value of types of counselling and the skills of counsellors.

What is the case against?

- ✓ It has been said that doctors may avoid contact with difficult patients by referring.
- ✓ Patients may therefore feel rejected in some cases and fail to attend.
- ✓ Some patients may feel worse after counselling.
- ✓ Financial costs are sometimes prohibitive and nationally the service offered on the NHS is patchy.

CHAPTER 5:
THE ELDERLY

CHAPTER 5:
THE ELDERLY

National Service Framework (NSF) for older people

The NSF is a 10-year strategy to ensure fair, high-quality integrated health and social care services for older people. It is designed to support independence and to promote good health.

The four themes in the NSF are:

1. Respecting the individual

2. Intermediate care

3. Providing evidence-based specialist care

4. Promoting an active, healthy life.

The NSF has eight standards

Standard 1: Rooting out age discrimination

NHS services will be provided, regardless of age, on the basis of clinical need alone. Social care services will not use age in their eligibility criteria or policies, to restrict access to available services.

Standard 2: Person-centred care

NHS and social care services should treat older people as individuals and enable them to make choices about their own care. This can be achieved through the single assessment process, integrated commissioning arrangements and integrated provision of services, including community equipment and continence services.

Standard 3: Intermediate care

Older people have access to a new range of intermediate care services at home or in designated care settings, to promote their independence by providing enhanced services from the NHS and councils to prevent unnecessary hospital admission and effective rehabilitation services to enable early discharge from hospital and to prevent premature or unnecessary admission to long-term residential care.

Intermediate care is a new layer of care, between primary care and specialist services. It is designed to prevent unnecessary hospital admission, support early discharge and reduce or delay long-term residential care. Sixty-three per cent of older people entering permanent nursing home care and 43% of those entering residential care homes come direct from hospital.

Standard 4: General hospital care

Older people's care in hospital must be delivered through appropriate specialist care (eg multidisciplinary teams headed by geriatricians) and by hospital staff who have the right set of skills to meet their needs.

Standard 5: Stroke (see Chapter 1, Cardiovascular Disease)

The NHS will take action to prevent strokes, working in partnership with other agencies where appropriate. People who are thought to have had a stroke must have access to diagnostic services and be treated appropriately by a specialist stroke service, and subsequently, with their carers, participate in a multidisciplinary programme of secondary prevention and rehabilitation.

Standard 6: Falls

The NHS will take action to prevent falls and reduce resultant fractures or other injuries in their populations of older people. Older people who have fallen must receive effective treatment and rehabilitation and, with their carers, receive advice on prevention, through a specialised falls service.

Standard 7: Mental health in older people

Older people who have mental health problems should have access to integrated mental health services, provided by the NHS and councils to ensure effective diagnosis, treatment and support, for them and for their carers.

Standard 8: The promotion of health and active life in older age

The health and well-being of older people is promoted through a co-ordinated programme of action led by the NHS with support from councils.

Falls

Fourteen thousand people die every year from osteoporotic hip fractures. Residents of nursing homes are at particularly high risk of falling and of having an adverse outcome from the fall.

Falling is often a result of an inadequately treated organic illness and can have potentially disastrous consequences, in terms of psychological morbidity (with the resulting lack of self confidence) and physical disability, both of which can lead to loss of independence.

One randomised controlled trial (RCT) found that chronic diseases and multiple pathology (including circulatory disease, chronic obstructive pulmonary disease, depression and arthritis) are more important predictors of falling than polypharmacy (*BMJ* 2003; **327**: 712–717).

A systematic review found that a multifactorial falls risk assessment and management programme was the most effective method of preventing further falls (*BMJ* 2004; **328**: 680).

NICE guidance, January 2004

All elderly people should be asked about whether they have fallen recently.

If they have, or they are considered to be at 'high risk', they should be assessed for gait and balance and whether they would benefit from any therapeutic intervention.

Patients specifically presenting after a fall, patients who report recurrent falls in the past year and patients with specific abnormalities of gait or balance should have a multifactorial falls assessment for which they may need to be referred to a falls clinic.

Any elderly patient being discharged from hospital should have input from an occupational therapist.

Elderly patients on psychotropic medication should have this gradually withdrawn if possible.

Home-based strength and balance training is recommended.

Psychological factors should be taken into account, such as fear of falling. The health care professional should ask specifically what actions the patient is prepared to take to reduce the risk of future falls.

Population approach to falls prevention

The incidence and impact of falls could be reduced through encouraging appropriate weight-bearing and strength-enhancing physical activity, promoting healthy eating and smoking cessation.

A community strategy to prevent falls should also include:

- ✓ Keeping pavements clear and in good repair.

- ✓ Adequate street lighting.

- ✓ Providing information, such as 'Avoiding Slips, Trips and Broken Hips' by the Department of Trade and Industry (DTI).

- ✓ Making property safer.

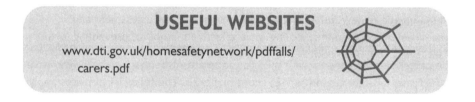

USEFUL WEBSITES

www.dti.gov.uk/homesafetynetwork/pdffalls/
carers.pdf

Depression

Numerous studies have demonstrated a community prevalence of depression in older people of 10–15% throughout the world.

Severe/psychotic depression has a prevalence of 1–3%. The prevalence of depression is much higher in nursing and residential homes at 22–33%.

Depression significantly affects quality of life and may adversely affect physical health. It can be triggered by a variety of factors, such as bereavement, life changes (eg retirement) and social isolation. Older people can also become depressed because of increasing illness or frailty, or following a stroke or a fall. Early recognition can reduce distressing symptoms and prevent physical illness, adverse effects upon social relationships, self-neglect and self-harm or suicide.

There is some evidence that depression is linked to cardiovascular morbidity. One study found that 12% of over 85-year-olds were depressed (*Int J Ger Psychiatry* 2004; **19**: 852–857). None were on antidepressants. When followed-up, the depressed subjects had double the cardiovascular mortality of non-depressed subjects.

Alzheimer's disease

Dementia affects 5% of people over the age of 65 years and 20% of people over the age of 80 years in the UK.

The three most common causes of dementia in the UK are Alzheimer's disease (accounts for 55% of cases), vascular dementia (25%) and Lewy body dementia (10–15%). Alzheimer's disease is characterised by a long preclinical period during which subtle cognitive deficits are often detectable.

Acetylcholinesterase inhibitors

The three drugs in this class are donepezil (Aricept®), galantamine (Reminyl®) and rivastigmine (Exelon®). All of them cost between £60 and £90 per month, depending on the dose prescribed. NICE have estimated that the NHS will spend more than £70m on cholinesterase inhibitors in 2005–6.

Side-effects are uncommon.

In their 2001 guidance, NICE recommends that the cholinesterase inhibitors can be prescribed for patients with mild to moderate Alzheimer's disease who have a mini mental state exam (MMSE) score of 12–26. The following provisos apply:

- ✓ Diagnosis and assessment of cognitive, global and behavioural functioning should take place in a specialist clinic and treatment must be initiated there.

- ✓ The drugs should be prescribed initially on a trial basis for 3–6 months. Only 'responders' should continue the drug, with response principally defined as no deterioration on MMSE score after 3–6 months.

- ✓ The patient should be followed up regularly and the cholinesterase inhibitor should only be continued if their MMSE does not deteriorate or drop to <12.

Cholinesterase inhibitors are not licensed for vascular dementia.

NICE came under a barrage of criticism when new draft guidance was published suggesting that these drugs are not cost-effective and should therefore no longer be initiated for dementia. NICE has partially reversed this controversial draft recommendation. Cholinesterase inhibitors should be considered in the treatment of patients with moderately severe disease but not for those with milder symptoms, according to the revised draft NICE guidance issued in January 2006.

Evidence

A meta-analysis of 10 trials involving 2376 patients given donepezil or placebo showed benefits in the donepezil group after 24 weeks (*Int J Ger Psychiatry* 2004; **19**: 624–633). Clinical evidence has concluded that donepezil and galantamine are likely to be beneficial (see box below).

 AD2000 (*Lancet* 2004; **363**: 2105)

✓ 565 community resident patients with mild to moderate Alzheimer's disease.

✓ Randomly allocated to donepezil or placebo for 12 weeks; 468 patients completed this period and were then re-randomised to placebo or to donepezil.

✓ Primary endpoints were entry to institutional care and progression of disability according to the Bristol activities of daily living scale (BADLS).

✓ The MMSE scores of patients treated with donepezil improved by an average of 0.8 and the BADLS score by 1.0 over the first 2 years.

✓ There was no benefit in donepezil over placebo in terms of institutionalisation, or in terms of behavioural and psychological symptoms, carer psychopathology, formal care costs, unpaid caregiver time, adverse events or deaths.

✓ The methodology has been criticised (eg the high drop out rates).

Another recent study set in the USA studied 769 patients with mild cognitive impairment, who were randomised to donepezil 10 mg, high-dose vitamin E or placebo and followed up for 3 years (*N Engl J Med* 2005; **352**: 2379–2388). Of the 769 patients 212 progressed to probable Alzheimer's disease over the course of the study. There was no significant difference in incidence of Alzheimer's disease between the three groups studied, although donepezil did appear to have a protective effect for the first 12 months compared to placebo (16 cases of Alzheimer's disease in the donepezil group in the first 12 months compared to 38 cases in the placebo group); however, this effect had disappeared by three years. Vitamin E was not found to be beneficial.

However, a recent systematic review of 22 RCTs has actually shown that the scientific basis for recommendations of cholinesterase inhibitors for the treatment of Alzheimer's is questionable (*BMJ* 2005; **331**: 321). Although the outcomes measuring cognition did show beneficial effects of cholinesterase inhibitors, these effects were minimal (ranging from 1.5 points to 3.9 points on a 70-point Alzheimer's disease assessment scale). It found that the methodological quality of the available trials was poor and benefits measured on rating scales were minimal.

Ginkgo biloba

A Cochrane review looked at the efficacy and safety of ginkgo use in patients with cognitive decline or dementia (*Cochrane Library*, Issue 2, Oxford, 2003):

No significant difference was found between ginkgo and placebo in terms of adverse events.

There was evidence of improvement in mood, cognition, activities of daily living and emotional function.

However, some of the newer trials included in the review showed inconsistent results and the authors stated that they could not rule out publication bias; larger trials are needed to clarify the situation.

Ginkgo is generally safe when used with low-dose (75 mg) aspirin, but should be avoided in patients on warfarin.

Clinical evidence 2005

- Beneficial — Donepezil, galantamine
- Likely to be beneficial — Memantine, ginkgo, reality orientation
- Trade-off between benefits and harms — Rivastigmine, tacrine
- Unknown effectiveness — Music therapy, NSAIDs, physostigmine, selegiline, reminiscence therapy
- Unlikely to be beneficial — Oestrogen

NMDA receptor antagonists

Glutamate neurones become inefficient in Alzheimer's disease, due to leakage at the *N*-methyl-D-aspartate (NMDA) receptor. This interferes with the transmission of the glutamate signal and can affect cognitive function. Memantine is an uncompetitive NMDA receptor antagonist and protects neurones from the toxic effects of elevated glutamate. Memantine is thought to be effective in moderate to severe Alzheimer's disease, as opposed to the cholinesterase inhibitors which can only be used in mild to moderate disease. It is sometimes used in combination with a cholinesterase inhibitor, either at the start of treatment or as the patient gets worse.

Other treatments

✓ Statins and NSAIDs: there has been much observational data about these drugs but not much in the way of hard evidence.

✓ Sensory stimulation: aromatherapy and bright light therapy may be effective in reducing restlessness and sleep disturbance in patients with Alzheimer's disease, with far fewer side-effects than sedative medication!

Drug treatment for disruptive features in dementia

Patients with advanced dementia may become increasingly aggressive or agitated. Symptoms which are present for more than 3 months are likely to persist long term.

Sedative medication is often prescribed because it makes life easier for the patient's carers; unfortunately, it is rarely in the best interests of the patient to be sedated and most of the available drugs have significant side-effects. In March 2004, the Committee on the Safety of Medicines (CSM) issued a warning about using atypical antipsychotics such as risperidone and olanzapine in patients with dementia; their use appears to be associated with a threefold increase in the risk of stroke. Although this risk has only been demonstrated with risperidone and olanzapine, it may also apply to other atypical antipsychotics.

The CSM recommendations are listed below:

Risperidone or olanzapine should not be used for the treatment of behavioural symptoms of dementia.

Use of risperidone for the management of acute psychotic conditions in elderly patients who also have dementia should be limited to the short-term and should be guided by specialist advice (olanzapine is not licensed for management of acute psychoses).

Prescribers should consider carefully the risk of cerebrovascular events before treating any patient who has a previous history of stroke or transient ischaemic attack with atypical antipsychotics. Consideration should also be given to other risk factors for cerebrovascular disease including hypertension, diabetes, current smoking and atrial fibrillation.

As always, nothing is ever straightforward in medicine. A population-based retrospective cohort study compared the incidence of admissions to hospital for stroke among older adults with dementia receiving atypical or typical antipsychotics (*BMJ* 2005; **330**: 445–448). In all, there were 32,710 participants, all ≥65 years, 17,845 of whom were on an atypical antipsychotic and 14,865 of whom were on a typical antipsychotic. Patients were observed until they were admitted to hospital with ischaemic stroke, stopped taking antipsychotics, died or the study ended. There was no significant increase in the risk of ischaemic stroke in the atypical antipsychotic group compared to the typical antipsychotic group.

Other potential treatment options include the conventional antipsychotics such as chlorpromazine, benzodiazepines (not recommended for long-term use), antidepressants and carbamazepine. There is only limited evidence supporting the use of carbamazepine, and treatment benefits will probably take at least three weeks to become apparent.

One recent trial showed that neither quetiapine nor rivastigmine is effective at reducing agitation at either 6 weeks or 26 weeks (*BMJ* 2005; **330**: 874–877). Quetiapine was associated with significantly greater cognitive decline than placebo at 6 weeks and 26 weeks.

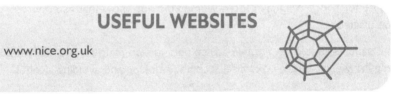

USEFUL WEBSITES

www.nice.org.uk

SUMMARY POINTS FOR ALZHEIMER'S DISEASE

✓ Dementia is very common

✓ Cholinesterase inhibitors may be less effective than initially thought

✓ NICE guidelines may change in the near future

Osteoporosis

Osteoporosis is defined as a skeletal disease characterised by low bone mass and deterioration of the microarchitecture of bone tissue, which makes bone more fragile and hence increases the risk of fracture.

Osteoporosis affects approximately 30% of women over the age of 80 in England and Wales. This is especially concerning given that, it is estimated, by 2025 almost a quarter of the population in Europe will be over 65. It is emerging as one of the biggest health problems in postmenopausal women, with one in three women over the age of 50 expected to sustain an osteoporotic fracture at some time in their life. Osteoporosis results in more deaths in older women than cancers of the cervix, uterus and ovaries combined. The annual cost to the NHS of osteoporotic fractures has been estimated at £1.7 billion; each hip fracture costs about £20,000. Approximately 20% of patients die within a year of sustaining a fractured neck of femur.

A low level of awareness of the benefits of early identification of risk factors, together with the pressure to reduce prescribing costs, often results in ineffective management. 'The Women's Health Report' was produced in February 2003 by the National Osteoporosis Society. This looked at women's knowledge of osteoporosis-related issues. Despite the fact that one in three women over the age of 50 years will be affected by osteoporosis, only 27% thought this was cause for concern. One in three women did not know that osteoporosis could be treated.

All patients should get lifestyle advice on nutrition (calcium and vitamin D), regular weight-bearing exercise, stopping smoking and avoiding alcohol.

The National Service Framework (NSF) for older people addresses the need for action on the prevention and treatment of osteoporosis. It also acknowledges that preventing osteoporosis in high-risk patients has a significant effect on both the number and severity of fractures.

 NICE guidance on treatment

NICE issued guidance for the secondary prevention of osteoporotic fractures in postmenopausal women in 2005.

The NICE recommendations are:

1. All women aged 75 years and over who have sustained an osteoporotic fragility fracture should be treated for presumed osteoporosis without need for a DEXA bone scan.

2. All women aged between 65 and 74 who have had an osteoporotic fracture should be treated if osteoporosis (defined as a T-score less than -2.5 SD) is confirmed by DEXA. If the wait for a DEXA scan is likely to be very long, treatment can be initiated while the patient is waiting and then modified according to the result of the scan.

3. Postmenopausal women younger than 65 years of age should be treated:

   a. if they have a very low bone mineral density (approximately -3 SD or below)

   b. if they have a bone mineral density (BMD) <-2.5 SD plus one or more additional risk factors:

      i.   low body mass index (<19 kg/m^2)

      ii. family history of maternal hip fracture before the age of 75 years

      iii. untreated premature menopause

      iv. medical disorders associated with bone loss (chronic inflammatory bowel disease, rheumatoid arthritis, hyperthyroidism, coeliac disease)

      v.   conditions associated with prolonged immobility.

For treatment, NICE guidance recommends the bisphosphonates (alendronate, etidronate and risedronate). Raloxifene is recommended as an alternative treatment option in women for whom bisphosphonates are ineffective or contraindicated or who are physically unable to comply with the recommendations for their use. Calcium and/or vitamin D supplementation should be provided to all women unless clinicians are confident that they have an adequate calcium intake and are vitamin D replete.

Teriparatide should be restricted for secondary prevention in women aged 65 years or older who have had an unsatisfactory response to bisphosphonates and:

   ✓ who have a T-score approximately -4 SD or below

   ✓ who have a T-score of approximately -3 SD or below with

      • multiple fractures or

      • one or more of the risk factors detailed above.

Some experts have challenged this NICE guidance as being unnecessarily restrictive to young women.

Primary prevention of osteoporosis

NICE also released draft guidance for the primary prevention of osteoporosis in postmenopausal women in 2005, ie where osteoporosis has been diagnosed, but where the woman has not yet sustained a fracture.

Bisphosphonates are recommended for the primary prevention of osteoporotic fragility fractures in the following groups of women:

✓ in women aged 70–74 years

- if they have one clinical risk factor and a *T*-score of –3.5 SD or below, or

- if they have two clinical risk factors and a *T*-score of –3 SD or below, or

- if they have three or more clinical risk factors and a *T*-score of –2.5 SD or below

✓ in women aged 75 years and over

- if they have one clinical risk factor and a *T*-score of –3 SD or below

- if they have two clinical risk factors and a *T*-score of –2.5 SD or below, or

- if they have three or more clinical risk factors, and in this case a DEXA scan is not necessary.

Strontium ranelate is recommended as an alternative treatment option in women:

✓ for whom bisphosphonates are contraindicated or who are unable to comply with the special instructions for the administration of bisphosphonates, or

✓ who are intolerant of bisphosphonates.

NICE does not recommend raloxifene for the primary prevention of osteoporotic fractures.

Strontium may be considered for secondary prevention when the guidance is rewritten in 2006.

Treatments for osteoporosis

Bisphosphonates

Bisphosphonates block osteoclast action. Cyclical etidronate, alendronate and risedronate are all licensed for the prevention and treatment of osteoporosis (and corticosteroid-induced osteoporosis).

The FACT study recently showed that alendronate once weekly improved bone mineral density at a significantly greater rate than risedronate once a week (*J Bone Miner Res* 2005; **20**: 141). A recent study is one of the first to report on (relatively) long-term use of alendronate (*N Engl J Med* 2004; **350**: 1189). Treatment with alendronate for 10 years led to impressive increases in bone mineral density. The safety data did not suggest that prolonged treatment was less beneficial.

Ibandronate (Boniva®) is an oral bisphosphonate. Whereas the other must be taken daily or weekly, ibandronate is taken only monthly. It is felt that this regime will limit adverse effects and improve compliance.

Absorption of all the bisphosphonates is very poor and tablets need to be taken on an empty stomach and food avoided for at least 30 minutes.

Selective oestrogen-receptor modulator therapy (SERMs)

Raloxifene mimics the beneficial effects of oestrogen on the bone but blocks the oestrogen effect on the uterus and breast tissue. It reduces vertebral fractures by 30% over 3 years, but does not reduce the incidence of non-vertebral fractures. It does not cause uterine bleeding or gastrointestinal side-effects, and reduces the risk of breast cancer; however, it worsens certain menopausal symptoms such as hot flushes and increases the risk of deep vein thrombosis (DVT).

Hormone-replacement therapy (HRT)

HRT is no longer recommended for primary or secondary prevention of osteoporosis (see Chapter 6, Obstetrics and Gynaecology) unless the patient is suffering from vasomotor symptoms.

Strontium ranelate

A new product, strontium ranelate (Protelos®) has recently been launched for postmenopausal women. It is a dual action bone agent, decreasing bone loss as well as increasing bone formation. The SOTI trial showed a 49% reduction in the incidence of new vertebral fractures in the first year (*N Engl J Med* 2004; **350**: 459). It is likely strontium will be used as an alternative for patients who cannot tolerate bisphosphonates (*Osteoporosis Rev* 2004; **12**: 8).

Calcium and vitamin D

Calcium and vitamin D supplements may slow down the rate of bone loss in elderly women who already have a low BMD and have been shown to reduce fractures, including hip fractures. However, in patients with established osteoporosis this effect is not enough. Calcium can however complement other treatments.

Vitamin D deficiency may contribute to osteoporosis and one study has concluded that if everyone over the age of 65 were routinely offered an oral vitamin D supplement (100,000 IU) every 4 months, then the rate of fractures could be reduced (*BMJ* 2003; **326**: 469). The NNT was found to be approximately 250 for 5 years to prevent one fracture and the benefit was more pronounced in women.

 The RECORD study (*Lancet* 2005; **365**: 1621–1628)

This was carried out in 21 centres in the UK and recruited 5292 healthy men and women living in the community (mean age 77) who had suffered a 'low-trauma' fracture. They were randomised to either vitamin D (800 IU per day), calcium (1000 mg per day), vitamin D and calcium or placebo. Active treatment failed to reduce fracture rates (including hip fracture), quality of life or survival over a 5-year follow-up period. However, the trial has been criticised for the following reasons:

✓ Of the 15,024 patients who would potentially have been eligible to take part in the trial, only 5292 were actually recruited.

✓ People who were eligible but who did not take part were older and were more likely to have suffered from hip fractures. It has been suggested that this group would derive most benefit from calcium and vitamin D supplements.

✓ Compliance was assessed using postal questionnaires and was poor (60% at 24 months among people who returned the questionnaire, or 47% overall, assuming that no one who failed to return the questionnaire was compliant).

Another study assessed 3314 women aged ≥70 years who had a clinical risk factor for hip fracture (*BMJ* 2005; **330**: 1003–1008). Its conclusion was that there was no evidence that calcium and vitamin D supplements reduce fracture rates. However, again compliance was poor, with only half the participants still taking medication at 24 months. Also, 48,987 women were invited to take part, of whom only 3314 agreed; this clearly leads to selection bias. Another potential source of bias is that the control group was given information on falls prevention and were advised on how to obtain sufficient vitamin D and calcium from dietary sources.

Calcitonin

This is an endogenous inhibitor of bone resorption, which suppresses osteoclasts. Salmon calcitonin (10 times more potent than human calcitonin) is available as a nasal spray and as a subcutaneous injection. It seems to have only a modest effect on bone density, but reduces the vertebral fracture rate by 33%.

Teriparatide

Teriparatide is a parathyroid hormone derivative. Studies have shown that it increases bone mineral density significantly more than alendronate (*J Bone Miner Res* 2003; **18**: 9) and leads to a lower incidence of fractures when compared with placebo (*Arch Intern Med* 2004; **164**: 2024). However, too few published studies have assessed teriparatide to define clearly what place, if any, it has in the management of osteoporosis.

Hip protectors

These seem to be effective in reducing the impact of falls when used properly, eg in institutionalised patients. However, in the community, compliance remains a huge problem.

Lifestyle factors

Encouraging people to cut down on smoking and alcohol, to eat a healthy diet and to do regular, weight-bearing or impact exercise can all help to reduce fracture rates.

USEFUL WEBSITES

www.doh.gov.uk/osteorep.htm – DoH guidelines on prevention and treatment (produced by the RCP)

www.nos.org.uk – National Osteoporosis Society

www.doh.gov.uk – National Service Framework for Older People

RISK FACTORS FOR OSTEOPOROSIS

✓ Early menopause

✓ Long-term prednisolone for ≥3 months

✓ Chronic disease (eg coeliac disease)

✓ Premenopausal episodes of amenorrhoea

✓ Lean body habitus

✓ Strong family history

✓ Cigarette smoking

SUMMARY POINTS FOR OSTEOPOROSIS

✓ Annual cost of osteoporosis to the NHS is £1.7 billion

✓ Often underdiagnosed and suboptimally managed

✓ Several effective medical interventions available

✓ Many patients are still not receiving treatment

✓ Bisphosphonates should be used first line

✓ Strontium seems a promising new treatment

✓ Poor compliance with treatment is a problem

Parkinson's disease

Parkinson's disease (PD) occurs worldwide with an equal incidence in men and women. Overall, age-adjusted prevalence is 1% worldwide (1.6% in Europe), rising from 0.6% at age 60–64, to 3.5% at age 85–89. The mean age of onset is 65. Onset can be insidious, and patients may simply present with recurrent falls and inability to cope.

PD is currently incurable and disability tends to be progressive. Treatment may slow down the rate of progression and reduce symptoms. In general, medication should be initiated by a neurologist or by a GP with a special interest in neurology.

Treatment options

Dopamine agonists (eg ropinirole, pramipexole, cabergoline, bromocriptine)

It is sometimes considered beneficial to start treatment with dopamine agonists instead of levodopa in early disease, especially in younger patients. Although dopamine agonists may not be as effective as levodopa (dopamine agonist monotherapy is associated with poorer motor scores than levodopa monotherapy and an increased risk of treatment withdrawal), they reduce the incidence of dyskinesias and fluctuations in motor response. Combination treatment can also reduce the risk of dyskinesia and may be used in late-stage PD. Longer-acting dopamine agonists such as ropinirole and pramipexole are less likely to induce dyskinesias than shorter-acting formulations.

Monoamine-oxidase-B inhibitors (eg selegiline)

A *Clinical Evidence* review in 2004 concluded that selegiline is beneficial in the early stages of PD and delays the need for levodopa compared to placebo. A recent meta-analysis also found that selegiline improves parkinsonian symptoms compared to placebo, delays the use of levodopa and is likely to be beneficial in patients with early disease (*BMJ* 2004; **329**: 593–596).

Levodopa (with dopa-decarboxylase inhibitor)

Although levodopa improves motor functioning, its use is associated in the long-term with dyskinesias and fluctuations in motor response that are irreversible. There is no benefit in taking modified-release preparations. Levodopa should be given with a dopa-decarboxylase inhibitor which reduces peripheral conversion of levodopa to dopamine, thus reducing adverse effects such as nausea.

Co-enzyme Q10

High-dose (1200 mg) co-enzyme Q10 seems to slow deterioration in the early stages of PD; at 18 months, one study showed a significant difference in functional status and disability (*Arch Neurol* 2002; **59**: 541). It is a very expensive treatment.

Deep brain stimulation

This may be helpful for severe dyskinesias.

Depression and PD

Depression is extremely common in PD; the global Parkinson Surveys estimate that up to 50% of patients are affected, although only 1% report their symptoms to a doctor. It is under-diagnosed, especially because sufferers often have a flat affect anyway, as a result of the disease. Patients who are treated with antidepressants are at risk of developing the serotonin syndrome, especially if they are already on selegiline. Selective serotonin-reuptake inhibitors (SSRIs) are probably the safest option (*BMJ* 2000; **320**: 1287).

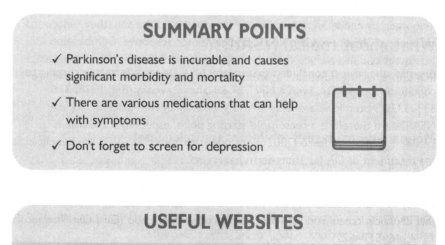

SUMMARY POINTS

✓ Parkinson's disease is incurable and causes significant morbidity and mortality

✓ There are various medications that can help with symptoms

✓ Don't forget to screen for depression

USEFUL WEBSITES

www.parkinsons.org.uk (website of the Parkinson's Disease Society, a UK charity dedicated to supporting people with Parkinson's, their families and carers)

www.clinicalevidence.com

Osteoarthritis

Osteoarthritis (OA) most commonly affects the hands, knees, hips and spine. It is a common and important cause of pain and disability, with about 10–20% of people over 60 years clinically affected, although radiographic changes in at least some joints are almost universal. The annual GP consultation rate is approximately 24.8/1000 for OA alone, and it accounts for 11% of all working days lost. The annual cost in the UK is estimated to be about £1.2 billion.

What is the evidence for glucosamine?

Glucosamine is claimed to have chondro-protective properties and is naturally occurring. There is evidence for its use, but this remains controversial; different RCTs have come to different conclusions.

In 2004, clinical evidence found limited evidence that glucosamine was more effective than placebo in improving pain and function in people with OA of the knee; a systematic review found limited evidence that glucosamine improved pain symptoms compared with NSAIDs (*The Cochrane Library*, Issue 2 2004). Glucosamine was found to be as safe as placebo and less likely than NSAIDs to produce adverse events. Glucosamine is available on FP10, but is rarely prescribed, maybe due to a lack of clear guidelines and concerns about cost.

What about topical NSAIDs?

A systematic review concluded that topical NSAIDs are effective in chronic pain conditions such as OA, with a NNT of 3.1 after 2 weeks (*BMJ* 1998; **316**: 333–337). Systemic side-effects are no greater than with placebo. Topical NSAIDs are therefore a reasonable starting point, especially if the pain is localised. *Clinical Evidence* (2002) concludes that topical NSAIDs are beneficial in the treatment of OA for short-term pain relief.

Topical capsaicin cream may be an effective alternative for some patients. One non-systematic meta-analysis of three RCTs of topically applied capsaicin found that capsaicin cream reduced pain compared with placebo (*Eur J Clin Pharmacol* 1994; **46**: 517–522).

Who should be on cyclo-oxygenase-2 (COX-2) inhibitors?

COX-2 inhibitors are thought to offer a degree of gastrointestinal (GI) protection compared to NSAIDs; 10–20% of those taking long-term conventional NSAIDs develop gastric or duodenal ulcers detected endoscopically and 20–40% have mucosal erosions. Severe GI toxicity from NSAIDs accounts for 700–2000 deaths per annum in UK.

The incidence of endoscopic ulceration and erosions with COX-2 inhibitors is only 5–7% (*Drug Ther Bull* 2005; **43**(1)).

NICE 2001 guidance states that COX-2 inhibitors are not recommended for routine use in patients with rheumatoid arthritis or OA but should be used only in patients who are at 'high risk' of developing serious GI adverse effects.

These patients include those of 65 years of age and over, those using concomitant medications known to increase the likelihood of upper GI adverse events (not including aspirin), those with serious co-morbidity and those requiring the prolonged use of maximum recommended doses of standard NSAIDs.

However, there have been major concerns about cardiovascular safety with these drugs. Controversy over the cardiovascular effects of the COX-2 inhibitors has increased since the publication of the VIGOR study (*N Engl J Med* 2000; **343**: 1520). This suggested that taking rofecoxib increased the risk of future myocardial infarction. The APPROVe study led to the withdrawal of Vioxx® as the incidence of cardiovascular events was double with rofecoxib compared to placebo (*N Engl J Med* 2005; **352**: 1092).

A pooled analysis of the cardiovascular safety of several COX-2 inhibitors in a high-risk population did not provide any evidence of an increased risk (*Arch Intern Med* 2005; **165**: 181).

Studies have shown that celecoxib does not increase the morning or the 24-h average blood pressure in patients with controlled hypertension (*Hypertension* 2004; **43**: 573). However, a recent meta-analysis of the effects of COX-2 inhibitors on blood pressure pooled data on the risk of new-onset hypertension and found that COX-2 inhibitors were more likely to produce a significant rise in blood pressure than conventional NSAIDs (*Arch Intern Med* 2005; **165**: 1).

The European medicines agency (EMEA) subsequently reviewed the safety of the COX-2 inhibitors celecoxib, etoricoxib, lumiracoxib, parecoxib and valdecoxib in 2005. They issued the following recommendations:

1. COX-2 inhibitors must not be used in patients with established ischaemic heart disease, cerebrovascular disease or peripheral arterial disease.

2. Healthcare professionals are advised to exercise caution when prescribing COX-2 inhibitors to patients with risk factors for heart disease, such as hypertension, hyperlipidaemia, diabetes and smoking.

3. COX-2 inhibitors should be used at the lowest effective dose for the shortest possible duration of time.

4. The balance of cardiovascular and gastrointestinal risks should be carefully considered for patients who do not have heart disease but are taking low-dose aspirin. Evidence suggests that any gastrointestinal safety advantage for COX-2 inhibitors is substantially reduced when given with aspirin (NICE does not recommend the use of a COX-2 inhibitor in conjunction with aspirin).

The EMEA also recommended that valdecoxib should have its marketing authorisation suspended.

What about NSAIDs and cardiovascular risk?

Most data suggest that conventional NSAIDs either have no impact on the risk of cardiovascular events, or may even be cardioprotective (although to a lesser extent than aspirin) (*Br J Cardiol* 2005; **12**: 387).

The Medicines and Healthcare products Regulations Agency (MHRA) published a report in August 2005 that considered the cardiovascular safety of traditional NSAIDs (www.mhra.gov.uk). Its conclusion was that the evidence of an increased thrombotic risk with NSAIDs is much less clear than for COX-2 inhibitors. The available evidence was considered inadequate to allow firm conclusions to be drawn about any increased risk of cardiovascular disease with NSAIDs, or to confidently differentiate between the risks of individual products. Based on the available evidence, it was thought that any increased risk is likely to be small and associated with continuous longer-term treatment and high doses.

Most of the available data relate to naproxen, ibuprofen and diclofenac. Some trials have shown naproxen to have a lower thrombotic risk than the COX-2 inhibitors. However, information on the risk for ibuprofen and diclofenac compared to COX-2 inhibitors is less clear.

Overall, the existing data were thought to be insufficient to warrant changes in current prescribing practice. All NSAIDs should be used at the lowest effective dose and for the shortest period of time necessary to control symptoms.

Other treatments

✓ **Intra-articular hyaluronic acid injections**; this seems to reduce pain in the short-term. *Clinical Evidence* (2002) concludes that hyaluronic acid is 'likely to be beneficial'.

✓ **Arthroplasty.** There is no doubt that joint replacement is effective; hip replacement is effective for at least 10 years. However, patients over 75 or under 45 and obese patients may have worse outcomes. Computer navigation is said to improve accuracy of prosthesis placement, which should in turn improve longevity.

✓ **Hip resurfacing.** There has been much publicity in the lay press regarding the 'Birmingham resurfacing hip replacement', where only the arthritic joint surface is replaced, preserving much of the femoral head. Although this has many theoretical advantages, especially in the younger patient, there are few valid long-term data as yet.

✓ **Unicompartmental knee replacement** is another less aggressive option, where only the damaged femoro-tibial compartment is replaced. This can be useful in the younger patient as it can be revised to a total knee replacement years later. It is an alternative to the older option of tibial osteotomy in varus knee OA, although tibial osteotomy is also making a bit of a comeback in the management of varus knee OA in a patient too young for total knee replacement.

✓ **Arthroscopic debridement** of the knee is another 'time buying measure', but the results (50% improvement in symptoms) are the same result as sham arthroscopy!

✓ **Minimal access arthroplasty** is currently very trendy and is popular in the private sector, but the jury is still out as to its usefulness over more established open techniques.

✓ **Artificial disc replacement** is increasingly used as an alternative to spinal fusion in the neck or lumbar spine. There are still no long-term results, but NICE have recently approved the technique for use in limited situations.

✓ **Taping of the knee joint.** Australian researchers have recently shown that therapeutic taping of the knee joint reduces short-term pain and disability compared to placebo (*BMJ* 2003; **327**: 135–138). This is not widely done in the UK.

✓ **Autologous chondrocyte transplantation.** This relatively new treatment is most useful in younger patients with a focal area of cartilage loss. Chondrocytes are harvested from the patient and multiplied in the lab, before being re-introduced arthroscopically, in an attempt to correct the cartilage defect.

✓ **Physiotherapy, weight loss** (hugely important)**, exercises eg quad strengthening, regular simple analgesia.**

SUMMARY POINTS

✓ OA is common

✓ Glucosamine is of uncertain benefit

✓ The future of COX-2 inhibitors is uncertain

✓ Lifestyle factors are, as always, very important

✓ There are many surgical options besides traditional hip and knee replacements.

CHAPTER 6:
OBSTETRICS AND GYNAECOLOGY

CHAPTER 6:
OBSTETRICS AND GYNAECOLOGY

Hormonal contraception

The combined oral contraceptive pill (COCP)

About 80% of British women use the COCP at some time between the ages of 16 and 24 years.

What is the risk of deep vein thrombosis (DVT) in women taking the COCP?

Women with a body mass index (BMI) of ≥ 35 kg/m^2 have a fourfold increased risk of DVT when taking any type of combined oral contraceptive.

A meta-analysis in the *British Medical Journal* concluded that the DVT risk associated with a third-generation pill is 1.7 times that of a second-generation pill (*BMJ* 2001; **323**: 131–134).

The quoted risks of DVT per year are as follows:

Non-users	5:100,000
Second-generation pill	15:100,000
Third-generation pill	30:100,000
Pregnancy	60:100,000

In 1999, the Department of Health announced an end to the 1995 restrictions on prescribing third-generation oral contraceptive pills. The absolute risk of venous thromboembolism (VTE) in women taking either second- or third-generation combined oral contraceptives remains very small and is still well below the risk associated with pregnancy. If VTE occurs at all, it is most likely to do so in the first year of treatment; risk is subsequently low. Provided that women are informed of and accept the relative risks of thromboembolism, the choice of oral contraceptive is for the woman and the prescriber to decide jointly, in the light of her individual medical history and any contraindications.

Is there an increased risk of myocardial infarction?

A recent large community-based case–control study found no association between use of the combined oral contraceptive and myocardial infarction, and no difference in risk between second- and third-generation pills (*BMJ* 1999; **318**: 1579–1584). Conversely, a meta-analysis of 14 studies found that the use of low-dose oral contraceptives was associated with a doubling of the risk of cardiovascular outcomes (myocardial infarction or ischaemic stroke) (*J Clin Endocrinol Metab* 2005; **90**: 3863). This meta-analysis found that although both second- and third-generation oral contraceptives were associated with a significantly increased risk of ischaemic stroke, the association between third-generation oral contraceptive use and myocardial infarction proved non-significant.

The risk of myocardial infarction in women taking the COCP seems to increase only in association with additional risk factors (eg smoking, diabetes, obesity, hypertension). The COCP is contraindicated in women with severe or multiple risk factors for ischaemic heart disease.

Does taking the COCP lead to hypertension?

There is a lack of data on the effects of the low-dose combined oral contraceptive on blood pressure. If a woman develops pill-induced hypertension, she should consider an alternative method of contraception. The pill is contraindicated in patients with a sustained blood pressure above 160/100 mmHg (or 140/90 mmHg in women over 35 years old).

Is the COCP contraindicated in women with migraine?

A potential association between the risk of stroke and migraine is an important public health concern, especially in young women who use oral contraceptives (*Contraception* 2002; **65**: 197).

It has previously been thought that taking the combined oral contraceptive, even in low dose, increases the risk of future stroke. However, in a pooled analysis involving more than one million people, it was found that there was no increased risk of stroke in women taking the oral contraceptive (*Arch Intern Med* 2004; **164**: 741).

The results of a recent systematic review and meta-analysis strongly suggest that migraine may be an independent risk factor for stroke (*BMJ* 2005; **330**: 63). The increased relative risks of ischaemic stroke were 1.8 in migraine without aura, 2.3 in migraine with aura and 8.7 in women with migraine who are taking the oral contraceptive pill. However, no distinction was made between users of oral contraceptive pills containing high doses of oestrogen and those containing low doses or only progesterone.

The COCP is contraindicated in patients who have migraines with aura (focal migraine) or frequent or severe migraines, those treated with ergot derivatives, those with migraines lasting for >72 h despite treatment and in women who have other strong risk factors for arterial disease.

What was the cervical cancer scare about?

Cervical cancer and the COCP systematic review
(*Lancet* 2003; **361:** 1159–1167)

Human papillomavirus (HPV) is thought to be the most important cause of cervical cancer. The COCP may increase the risk of cervical cancer in HPV-positive women. This systematic analysis looked at data from 28 studies (including 12,531 women) to examine the relationship between invasive and in situ cervical cancer and duration and frequency of use of hormonal contraceptives, with particular attention paid to HPV infection.

✓ The relative risks of cervical cancer increased with increasing duration of COCP use: for durations of <5 years, 5–9 years, and ≥10 years, respectively, the relative risks were 1.1, 1.6 and 2.2 for all women; and 0.9, 1.3 and 2.5 for HPV-positive women.

✓ The results were broadly similar for invasive and in situ cervical cancers, for squamous cell and adenocarcinoma, and in studies that adjusted for HPV status, number of sexual partners, cervical screening, smoking, or use of barrier contraceptives.

✓ The relative risk of cervical cancer may decrease after use of oral contraceptives ceases, but this is not certain from the limited data available.

✓ The Committee on the Safety of Medicines (CSM) have concluded that the overall risk is still very small and that women on the pill should simply be encouraged to have regular smears.

What about breast cancer?

There has recently been a large case–control study of 5000 women in America, which found no increase in the risk of breast cancer for current or previous use (*N Engl J Med* 2002; **346**: 2025). However, in women who are positive for the BRCA1 gene, it may be best avoided – smaller studies have shown that there is an increased risk in this case.

Are there benefits from taking the COCP?

It is important to remember that the pill has numerous advantages. These include:

- ✓ Excellent efficacy and acceptability
- ✓ Beneficial effects on menstrual disorders
- ✓ Suppression of benign breast disease
- ✓ Protection against endometrial and ovarian cancer
- ✓ Protection against pelvic inflammatory disease.

Newer alternatives to the COCP

Evra®
This is a contraceptive patch releasing 20 micrograms per day of oestradiol and 150 micrograms of norelgestromin (the primary active metabolite in Cilest®). One review showed that Evra® is as effective as the COCP, but compliance is better (*JAMA* 2001; **285**: 2347–2354). It is more expensive than the COCP, and may not be effective in women weighing >90 kg.

NuvaRing®
This is a contraceptive vaginal ring containing 15 micrograms ethinyloestradiol and 120 micrograms etonogestrel.

The progesterone only pill (POP)
Cerazette® is a relatively new POP, containing a higher dose of progestogen than conventional POPs. It is thought to inhibit ovulation, and may have a similar efficacy to the COCP. It is the only POP with a 12-h missed pill window; the other formulations available have only a 3-h window. Barrier contraception needs to be used for 2 days following a missed pill. If unprotected intercourse took place during this period, then use of the emergency contraceptive pill should also be considered.

Depot progesterones

Depo-Provera® is a highly reliable form of contraception, the pregnancy rate being less than 4 per 1000 women treated for 2 years. On average, it takes 5 months for fertility to return to normal after use is stopped. Because of its effects on reducing bone mineral density (BMD), the CSM recommends reviewing women every 2 years to assess whether the benefits still outweigh the risks. Most of the reduction in BMD occurs in the first 2–3 years of use and then stabilises, with a probable return to normal after use stops.

The CSM recommends that Depo-Provera® should only be used as a first-line contraceptive in adolescents if other methods are unacceptable, and that women with risk factors for osteoporosis (eg heavy smoking, anorexia, long-term steroid use) should be advised to use alternative methods of contraception.

NICE guidance on long-acting reversible contraception (LARC) October 2005; Key points

Only about 8% of women aged 16–49 in the UK use LARC, compared with 25% who use the oral contraceptive pill and 23% who use male condoms.

- ✓ Women requiring contraception should be given information about, and offered a choice of, LARC as well as other methods.

- ✓ All currently available LARC methods (intrauterine devices, the intrauterine system, injectable contraceptives and implants) are more cost-effective than the combined oral contraceptive pill even at 1 year of use.

- ✓ Intrauterine devices, the intrauterine system and implants are more cost-effective than injectable contraceptives.

- ✓ Increasing the uptake of LARC methods is likely to reduce the numbers of unintended pregnancies.

- ✓ Women considering LARC should be given detailed verbal and written information, to help them to make an informed choice.

USEFUL WEBSITES

www.fpa.org.uk – Family Planning Association

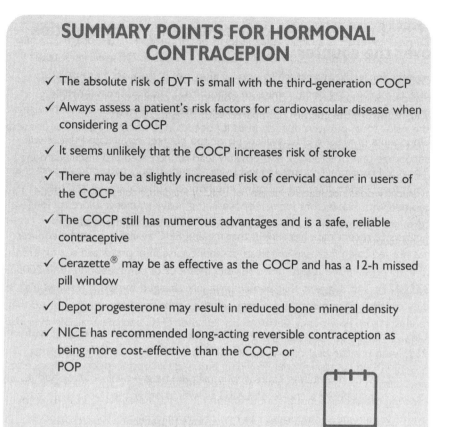

SUMMARY POINTS FOR HORMONAL CONTRACEPION

✓ The absolute risk of DVT is small with the third-generation COCP

✓ Always assess a patient's risk factors for cardiovascular disease when considering a COCP

✓ It seems unlikely that the COCP increases risk of stroke

✓ There may be a slightly increased risk of cervical cancer in users of the COCP

✓ The COCP still has numerous advantages and is a safe, reliable contraceptive

✓ Cerazette® may be as effective as the COCP and has a 12-h missed pill window

✓ Depot progesterone may result in reduced bone mineral density

✓ NICE has recommended long-acting reversible contraception as being more cost-effective than the COCP or POP

Emergency hormonal contraception

Emergency hormonal contraception (EHC) is a safe, cheap and highly effective way of preventing an accidental pregnancy. It is very popular; one-third of women aged 18–19 years and one-quarter of women aged 20–24 years have used it at least once over the preceding 2 years. Appropriate use of emergency contraception could prevent up to 75% of unplanned pregnancies.

Levonorgestrel is now the only available emergency contraception pill. A single dose of levonorgestrel 1.5 mg is as effective as the conventional doses of 750 micrograms according to a WHO trial in which over 4000 women in ten countries participated (*Lancet* 2002; **360**: 1803). In addition, it was found that extended use up to 120 h after intercourse does not cause an unacceptable deterioration in efficacy.

Use of progestogen-only emergency contraception over the counter

Over the counter EHC was legalised in 2001. A report from the Office for National Statistics says that 50% of women who obtained EHC in 2004–5 bought it from the chemist, compared with 27% in 2003–4.

Opponents of making EHC available over the counter have stated that it will encourage unprotected sex and possibly lead to increased promiscuity among teenagers (*N Engl J Med* 2003; **348**: 82). It has been shown that easier availability does not lead to 'abuse' of EHC (*J Paediatr Adolesc Gynecol* 2004; **17**: 87).

Analysis of recent data has shown that making EHC available over the counter has not led to an increase in its use, to an increase in unprotected sex or even to a decrease in the use of more reliable methods of contraception (*BMJ* 2005; **331**: 271). This suggests that people have just changed the place from which they obtain it. These results are supported by another study which showed that requests from emergency departments fell after EHC became available over the counter (*Emerg Med J* 2004; **21**: 67).

A randomised controlled trial providing emergency contraception in advance to post-partum women significantly increased the use of EHC without adversely affecting the use of routine contraception (*Obstet Gynecol* 2004; **102**: 8). In one study, women were randomised to one of pharmacy access to emergency contraception without a prescription, advance provision of emergency contraception, or usual care (requiring a visit to a clinic). Over the 6-month follow-up, women in the advance provision group were almost twice as likely to use emergency contraception than those in the other groups (*JAMA* 2005; **293**: 54). Furthermore, easier access to emergency contraception did not appear to affect regular contraceptive use or risky sexual behaviours.

USEFUL WEBSITES

www.ffprhc.org.uk – Faculty of Family Planning
and Reproductive Health Care

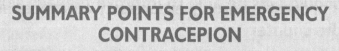

SUMMARY POINTS FOR EMERGENCY CONTRACEPION

✓ Emergency contraception is safe and cheap

✓ People from disadvantaged areas are less likely to take emergency contraception

✓ Easy access to EHC is effective

✓ Other forms of contraception are not affected by EHC use

✓ Levonorgestrel is obtainable without prescription

Teenagers and sexual health

The UK has the highest teenage pregnancy rate in Western Europe. Reduction in teenage pregnancy was one of the targets set for improvement during the 1990s in the Health of the Nation document; however it was not met!

What are the problems?

Teenagers are often confused about where they can obtain contraceptive advice or treatment, whether it is legal, whether it will be confidential and how to actually use the different contraceptive methods. The results of a questionnaire survey sent to 1045 children aged 13–15 years showed that 54% believed they had to be over 16 years of age to access sexual health services (*Br J Gen Pract* 2000; **50**: 550–554).

In the UK, approximately 50% of teenagers use contraception; this rate is much higher in Denmark, which suggests a poorer access and knowledge rather than lower demand in the UK. In addition, 75% of teenage mothers admit to having had unplanned pregnancies. However, figures released in April 2004 by the Office of National Statistics show that teenage conception rates have fallen for the third year in a row.

A report has found that women under the age of 18 who live in more deprived areas of Britain have higher rates of conception than women in wealthier areas but are less likely to opt for an abortion (*BMJ* 2004; **329**: 14).

How should GPs be able to improve teenage sexual health?

The Department of Health has updated their guidance on confidentiality when treating adolescents under the age of 16.

- ✓ Young people should be reassured that any doctor or nurse they see regarding sexual health matters will maintain confidentiality.

- ✓ It is recommended that clinics display their confidentiality policies clearly. If a doctor is not prepared to provide confidential services to young people under the age of 16, this should be advertised prominently along with information on alternative local services. Teenagers often prefer to seek help on contraceptive issues from a family planning clinic instead of from their GP.

- ✓ The doctor or nurse should discuss the emotional and physical implications of sexual activity with the young person and check that there is no element of coercion or abuse. They should be encouraged to confide in their parents.

To maximise the impact of services in promoting sexual health in adolescents, more innovative means of offering advice and promoting sexual health are needed (*BMJ* 2005; **330**: 107).

It is clear that GPs should follow-up teenage patients to ensure that they are using their contraception correctly. In addition, patients who receive emergency contraception should be started on regular contraception at the same time and then have clear follow-up arrangements.

Unfortunately, a recent systematic review concluded that primary prevention strategies have not actually been shown to delay the initiation of sexual intercourse or improve the use of contraception among teenagers (*BMJ* 2002; **324**: 1426–1429).

Confidentiality and teenage sex

The Fraser ruling has generally been used as the arbiter to clarify the legal position of treating children under the age of 16 without parental consent (see following box).

However, there has recently been concern about local guidelines issued by area child protection committees (including the pan-London committee) that call for the mandatory reporting of all sexually active children under the age of 13 to the police and Social Services, seemingly in direct contradiction of the Fraser ruling.

Doctors have also been instructed to ask the police whether they hold information about any sexually active 13 to 16 year olds and their partners. Although the police will not treat these requests as formal allegations of a crime, they will keep them on record. The legal standing of these protocols is unclear, and the British Medical Association, General Medical Council and Royal College of General Practitioners have signed a joint statement attacking them. Doctors who follow the protocols currently risk legal and professional action.

It has been estimated in various surveys that at least one-quarter of teenagers do not believe their consultation will be confidential, and such adverse publicity is unlikely to help the situation.

CONTRACEPTION AND YOUNG PEOPLE UNDER 16 YEARS – THE FRASER GUIDELINES

A young person under 16 years may be given advice and may be prescribed contraception without parental consent if the following conditions are met:

- ✓ They understand the advice and are competent to consent to treatment

- ✓ You encourage them to inform their parent(s) or guardian

- ✓ You believe they are likely to commence or continue sexual activity with or without contraception

- ✓ Their physical or mental health will suffer if they do not receive contraception advice or supplies

- ✓ Providing contraception is in their best interest

USEFUL WEBSITES

www.teenagepregnancyunit.gov.uk – Teenage Pregnancy Unit's website

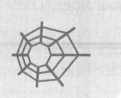

SUMMARY POINTS FOR TEENAGERS AND SEXUAL HEALTH

✓ The UK has a high teenage pregnancy rate

✓ Most teenagers are unaware of confidentiality issues and of the different contraceptive choices available

✓ Sexual health is important in teenagers

✓ Teenage pregnancy rates appear to be reducing

✓ Teenage health is often neglected

✓ GPs should be providing better health care for teenagers

Sexual health and chlamydia

The incidence of sexually transmitted infections (STIs) in the UK is rapidly rising, despite government initiatives such as the 'National strategy for sexual health and HIV' (2001). The UK teenage pregnancy rate is still the highest in Western Europe and only 50% of under 16s use contraception at first intercourse.

Chlamydia is the commonest curable sexually transmitted disease in the industrialised world and is currently a huge problem in young, sexually active adults; 36% of adults diagnosed with it are aged under 20. Chlamydia produces few or no symptoms in up to 70% of affected women and 50% of men. Around 15% of women may become infertile after a single episode of pelvic inflammatory disease (PID), 10% may develop chronic pelvic pain and 10% of subsequent pregnancies may be ectopic. Chlamydia has been implicated in 50% of cases of PID. The NHS spends £50 m a year treating infertility secondary to chlamydial infections.

Prevalence

Results from the national chlamydia screening programme in 2003–04 showed a prevalence of 10.1% for women and 13.3% for men under 25 years of age. Considerable rises in the incidence of chlamydia have led to a major public health problem in the UK (*BMJ* 2005; **330**: 590).

Chlamydia infections rose by 9% overall between 2002 and 2003. Between 1995 and 2003, they increased by 196% in men and by 188% in women (*BMJ* 2004; **329**: 249).

Data from the National Survey of Sexual Attitudes and Lifestyles were recently re-analysed to determine whether there is a difference between high-risk sexual behaviour and adverse sexual health outcomes amongst five different ethnic groups (*Lancet* 2005; **365**: 1246–1255); the conclusion was that although Afro-Caribbean and Black African men tended to have a higher number of sexual partners (median 9) than white men, this only went some way towards explaining the difference in STI incidence and could not explain it fully. White women reported a higher number of lifetime sexual partners (median 5) than black women (median 4) but black Afro-Caribbean women had a higher rate of STIs. Odds ratios changed little after controlling for age, number of sexual partnerships, homosexual and overseas partnerships and condom use at last sexual intercourse.

Number of adverse sexual health outcomes

	1995	2002	2003	2004
All STI diagnoses	428,575	703,525	735,302	751,282
Syphilis	102	1,258	1,641	2,252
Chlamydia	29,241	87,596	95,879	103,932
Gonorrhoea	9,950	25,599	24,915	22,320

Source: Health Protection Agency data

What is the independent advisory group for sexual health and HIV?

The independent advisory group (IAG) for sexual health and human immunodeficiency virus (HIV) was set up in 2003 to monitor the progress of the National Strategy for Sexual Health and HIV. In its first report in 2004, it made 29 recommendations including the following:

- ✓ Increased availability of free condoms and removal of value added tax (VAT) from over-the-counter contraceptives.

- ✓ NHS to fund at least 90% of abortions.

- ✓ Average wait for a genitourinary (GU) clinic to be no more than 48 h.

- ✓ Provision of sexual health services tailored to ethnic minority groups.

- ✓ Inclusion of sexual health services within the quality and outcomes framework (QOF).

National chlamydia screening programme (NCSP)

Although opportunistic chlamydia screening is being introduced in England, there is no high quality evidence of its effectiveness. The NCSP has been implemented by the Department of Health. Its goals are to:

✓ Control chlamydia through the early detection and screening of asymptomatic infection.

✓ To prevent the development of sequelae.

✓ To prevent onward transmission.

The slow progress of implementation of screening reflects the time taken to roll out this complex public health programme, in a considered manner, over 5 years. The scale of the exercise is considerable, given the unique nature of the programme, the range of sites being included, and the immense challenges of implementation in the context of a changing NHS (*BMJ* 2004; **329**: 172).

The specimens used in the screening programme will be:

✓ Urine specimens (male and female).

✓ Self taken vulvo-vaginal swabs.

✓ Endocervical swabs when a smear is being taken.

✓ Phased implementation started in England in 2002. National roll-out is expected by March 2007.

✓ The idea is to provide opportunistic testing for chlamydia in non-symptomatic, sexually active men and women who are under the age of 25 (including contacts of patients with confirmed STDs).

✓ Patients should be offered repeat testing according to their own individual risk, but usually there should be a minimum period of 5 weeks between tests.

✓ Testing is to be done in a variety of settings including primary care, family planning clinics, colposcopy units and termination of pregnancy clinics.

✓ Urine or self-collected vulvo-vaginal swabs are analysed using nucleic acid amplification technology (NAAT). NAAT is the most accurate method of detecting chlamydia, and the IAG has recommended that it should replace 'sub-optimal' non-molecular methods in a phased nationally rolled-out programme.

✓ It is likely that much of the work will be done in primary care and sexual health may be included as part of QOF in the future.

One study showed that a lack of willingness to discuss sexual health at unrelated consultations and a lack of time have resulted in many GPs not being completely involved with screening for chlamydia (*Br J Gen Pract* 2004; **54**: 508).

Is postal screening for chlamydia feasible? ClaSS (chlamydia screening studies) project (*BMJ* 2005; **330**: 940–943)

✓ 19,773 men and women aged 16–39, living in the West Midlands and Avon, selected at random from 27 general practices.

✓ Invited to collect their own specimens (urine for men and urine and vulvovaginal swab in women) and to complete a risk-assessment questionnaire. These then had to be posted back to the researchers.

✓ Samples were analysed using NAAT.

✓ 73% of patients were contactable.

✓ Uptake of screening was 34.5% overall, and 31.5% in 16- to 24-year-olds; sometimes a single postal invitation was insufficient, and patients needed further postal reminders or reminders by their GP. The authors conclude that repeated reminders had little impact on increasing uptake overall and would be unfeasible in routine practice.

✓ Uptake was lower in deprived areas. Young women at higher risk of infection were harder to engage in screening.

✓ The overall prevalence of chlamydia was 2.8% in men and 3.6% in women but these figures were higher in the 16- to 24-year-old age group (5.1% in men and 6.2% in women).

✓ The relatively modest uptake of screening and inaccuracies in demographic data held by general practices may limit the usefulness of postal screening.

STIs and social status (*Sex Transm Infect* 2005; **81**: 41–46)

This study was based in Leeds and examined risk factors for STIs. Age (15–24), ethnicity (Blacks>Whites>Asians) and residence in inner city areas of deprivation were found to be independent risk factors for chlamydia, *Gonorrhoea* and HPV. Seventy per cent of cases of chlamydia in the community could be detected by screening women <25 years.

Why has the incidence of STIs, including chlamydia, increased by so much?

Some of the rise in incidence may be a reflection of improved detection and awareness. However, one of the major factors is changing sexual behaviour. In addition, levels of awareness and fear of HIV have declined, and the major fear is now of unintended pregnancy (*BMJ* 2001; **322**: 1135–116).

USEFUL WEBSITES

www.doh.gov.uk – report of the Chief Medical Officer's expert advisory group on *Chlamydia*

www.chlamydia.ac.uk – *Chlamydia* screening studies (ClaSS) project

www.fpa.org.uk

SUMMARY POINTS FOR CHLAMYDIA

✓ *Chlamydia* is most prevalent sexually transmitted disease (STD) in the UK

✓ The highest rates are in females aged 16–24 years

✓ Most patients are asymptomatic

✓ The National Screening Programme is being implemented

✓ There is a continued lack of public awareness of *Chlamydia*

✓ Training and resources are a problem for screening

Hormone replacement therapy

Risks of hormone replacement therapy

There has been much adverse publicity recently about hormone replacement therapy (HRT) because of the results from two large studies which are detailed below. The situation is far from clear cut however; for example, a recent meta-analysis of 30 studies involving more than 26,000 women (*J Gen Intern Med* 2004; **19**: 791–804) showed that in women below the age of 60, using HRT reduces mortality by 40%. Although this benefit was not shown to extend to the >60 year age group, no overall increase in mortality was demonstrated in HRT users (including separate analyses for cardiovascular deaths and cancer-related deaths).

Fears about the risks of HRT have led to a substantial decline in its use (*Ann Intern Med* 2004; **140**: 184). A recent consensus statement (December 2004) from the Royal College of Obstetricians and Gynaecologists made the following recommendations:

- ✓ HRT should continue to be prescribed for women with severe menopausal symptoms.

- ✓ For women who are not suffering from menopausal symptoms, the risks of taking HRT outweigh the benefits.

- ✓ Ultimately women should have the choice of whether or not to take HRT, provided they understand the risks.

The largest risk factor for breast cancer in postmenopausal women is actually obesity – a woman with a BMI of >30 kg/m^2 has double the risk of breast cancer compared to a woman of normal weight. This is the same risk as is created by combined HRT or drinking more than two units of alcohol daily (*Lancet* 2003; **362**: 419).

A recent paper has worked out the cumulative absolute lifetime risks to individual women who take HRT up to the age of 79 (*BMJ* 2005; **331**: 347). Use of oestrogen-only hormone replacement or short-term (about 5 years) use of combined therapy starting at age 50 years hardly affects the cumulative breast cancer risk calculated to the age of 79 (no-use 6.1%, oestrogen-only 6.3%, combined 6.7%). Use of combined hormone replacement therapy for about 10 years increases the cumulative risk to 7.7%. These results are very reassuring.

☐ **Million Women Study (MWS)** (*Lancet* 2003; **362**: 419–427)

This was an observational study looking at the risk of breast cancer in nearly 1 million postmenopausal women living in the UK and taking various types of HRT over a 5-year period. The NHS Breast Screening Programme was used to recruit women.

The risk of breast cancer with use of HRT was found to be duration-dependent and declined once treatment was stopped, so that there was no excess risk after 5 years of being off HRT.

✓ The study found that women on combined HRT had double the risk of breast cancer compared to non-users; the increase in risk became apparent within 1–2 years of starting treatment.

✓ Women on oestrogen-only products had a relative risk of breast cancer of 1.3.

✓ Women on tibolone had a relative risk of breast cancer of 1.45.

✓ There was no evidence that different preparations of combined HRT resulted in different levels of risk.

✓ A more recent analysis of the MWS (*Lancet* 2005; **365**: 1543–1551) showed an increased risk of endometrial cancer in women on tibolone (relative risk, RR, 1.79) and oestrogen alone (RR 1.45). Women on continuous combined preparations had a lower risk of endometrial cancer (RR 0.71), but this did not apply to women on combined cyclical HRT (RR 1.05). The risks of tibolone and oestrogen alone were found to be greatest in non-obese women (obese women already have high levels of endogenous oestrogen in any case); conversely the protective effect of combined HRT was most pronounced in the obese.

✓ Despite the reduction in risk of endometrial cancer with continuous combined preparations, the overall cancer rate (ie combined breast and endometrial cancer rates) is still higher in women taking combined HRT (cyclical and continuous) than in women on oestrogen alone or tibolone.

The MWS was an observational study and its methodology has been criticised. For example, it may have underestimated the duration of usage of HRT, as it did not count years of HRT exposure from baseline (filling in of questionnaire) to breast cancer reporting on the UK cancer registry. Also, bearing in mind the natural history of breast cancer development, it is unlikely that the cancers diagnosed after 1 year had developed de novo – it is more likely that these cancers were missed by mammography at baseline and that HRT had acted as a promoter rather than an initiator.

Women's Health Initiative (WHI) Study (*JAMA* 2002; **288**: 321–333)

✓ This was a USA-based RCT that examined the risks and benefits of using a particular type of HRT (containing 0.625 mg conjugated equine oestrogens and 2.5 mg medroxyprogesterone acetate) in 16,608 long-term users, over 5.2 years (the intended duration of the study was 8.5 years, but it was stopped early due to a larger than expected number of breast cancer cases).

✓ It was thought at the time that HRT reduces the risk of cardiovascular disease (CVD), and the primary outcome in this trial was coronary heart disease (non-fatal myocardial infarction and coronary heart disease death), with invasive breast cancer as the primary adverse outcome.

✓ Critics have pointed out that the average age of enrolled women was 63, which is older than the average age of an HRT user in the UK.

Estimated hazard ratios with use of HRT were as follows: CHD 1.29; breast cancer 1.26; stroke 1.41; pulmonary embolism (PE) 2.13; colorectal cancer 0.63; endometrial cancer 0.83; hip fracture 0.66; and death due to other causes 0.92.

The absolute increases in risk per 10,000 women-years attributable to combined HRT were:

✓ 7 more CHD events (ie 3.5 extra cases per 1000 women treated for 5 years)

✓ 8 more strokes (ie 4 extra cases per 1000 women treated for 5 years)

✓ 8 more PEs (ie 4 extra cases per 1000 women treated for 5 years)

✓ 8 more invasive breast cancers (ie 4 extra cases per 1000 women treated for 5 years).

Absolute risk reductions per 10,000 women-years were:

✓ 6 fewer colorectal cancers (ie 3 fewer cases per 1000 women treated for 5 years)

✓ 5 fewer hip fractures (ie 2.5 fewer cases per 1000 women treated for 5 years)

Women's Health Initiative (WHI) Study – oestrogen-only arm (*JAMA* 2004; **291**: 1701–1712)

✓ 10,739 postmenopausal women, aged 50–79 years, with prior hysterectomy, including 23% of minority race/ethnicity.

✓ Women were randomly assigned to receive either 0.625 mg/day of oestrogen or placebo. The primary outcome was coronary heart disease (CHD) incidence (non-fatal myocardial infarction or CHD death). Again, invasive breast cancer incidence was the primary adverse outcome.

✓ Estimated hazard ratios after an average follow-up of 6.8 years were: CHD 0.91; breast cancer 0.77; stroke 1.39; PE 1.34; colorectal cancer 1.08; and hip fracture 0.61.

✓ Only the incidences of stroke and hip fracture were affected by oestrogen alone in a statistically significant manner; the absolute increase in risk of CVA equated to 12 additional strokes per 10,000 women-years. Conversely, there were 6 fewer hip fractures per 10,000 women-years. There was no increase in CHD and a possible reduction in breast cancer.

WHIMS (Women's Health Initiative Memory Study) (*JAMA* 2003;**289**: 2651–2662 and 2004; **291**: 2947–2958)

✓ These were separate branches of the Women's Health Initiative (WHI) looking at whether oestrogen alone or oestrogen plus medroxyprogesterone (MPA) alters global cognitive function in older women (aged 65–79 years).

✓ The primary endpoint was global cognitive function assessed annually by the modified mini-mental state examination.

✓ The mean follow-up period was 5.4 years.

✓ Incidence rates for probable dementia in the oestrogen-alone trial were statistically similar to those in the oestrogen plus progesterone trial (approximately 23 extra cases of dementia per 10,000 women years); the authors concluded that for women aged 65 years or older, hormone therapy had an adverse effect on cognition, which was greater among women with lower cognitive function at the initiation of treatment.

✓ The increase in absolute risk is small.

Meta-analysis of HRT and CVA risk (*BMJ* 2005; **330**: 342–344)

✓ 28 trials studied, including the WHI.

✓ 39,769 subjects.

✓ There was an increased risk of non-fatal ischaemic stroke (odds ratio, OR, 1.23, confidence interval, CI, 1.06–1.44).

✓ There was a non-significant trend towards increase in fatal stroke (OR 1.28, CI 0.87–1.88).

✓ Overall, there was a 29% increase in risk of stroke with use of HRT.

✓ No conclusions were drawn about whether oestrogen alone or transdermal preparations are safer.

NORA study (*Obstet Gynaecol* 2004; **103**: 440–446)

✓ Observational study of 140,584 women >50 years of age to assess whether HRT is protective against fractures.

✓ Started in 1997.

✓ 48% of women were on HRT at the start of the study.

✓ Only current users of HRT had a significantly different hip fracture rate.

NICE does not recommend HRT as a first-line treatment in the prevention or treatment of osteoporosis.

Breast cancer; CSM data

✓ The relative risk (RR) of breast cancer in women on combined HRT (compared to non-users) is approximately 2.00.

✓ The relative risk of breast cancer in women on tibolone is 1.45.

✓ The relative risk of breast cancer in women on oestrogen alone is 1.30.

✓ This extra risk of breast cancer becomes evident within 1–2 years of starting treatment.

✓ The extra risk of breast cancer starts to decline after a woman stops HRT and disappears altogether within 5 years after the HRT has been stopped.

✓ The extra risk of breast cancer does not apply to women prescribed HRT for premature ovarian failure; it only applies to postmenopausal women over the age of 50.

USEFUL WEBSITES

www.mhra.gov.uk information sheet for women about HRT

www.the-bms.org – British Menopause Society

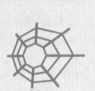

SUMMARY POINTS FOR HRT

✓ The Royal College of Obstetricians and Gynaecologists has issued a consensus statement regarding use of HRT

✓ HRT should only be used for symptomatic relief and not for disease prevention

✓ NICE does not recommend HRT as first line for osteoporosis prevention or treatment

✓ The excess risks associated with use of HRT do not apply to women under the age of 50

✓ Recent studies have provoked much anxiety in patients

✓ Risks of HRT need to be put into perspective

Table: Summary of risks associated with HRT

Disease	Extra number of cases per 1000 women using HRT for 5 years	Extra number of cases per 1000 women using HRT for 10 years
Breast cancer*	1.5 extra cases with oestrogen alone 6 extra cases with combined HRT	5 extra cases with oestrogen alone 19 extra cases with combined HRT
Endometrial cancer	4 extra cases with oestrogen alone Negligible risk with combined HRT	10 extra cases with oestrogen alone <2 with combined HRT
Ovarian cancer	1 extra case with oestrogen alone Negligible risk with combined HRT	3 extra cases with oestrogen alone Negligible risk with combined HRT
Stroke	1 extra case with oestrogen alone or combined HRT in women under 59 years 4 extra cases in women aged between 60 and 69 years	Data not available
Venous thrombo-embolism	4 extra cases with oestrogen alone or combined HRT in women under 59 years 9 extra cases in women aged between 60 and 69 years	Data not available

Table: Summary of benefits associated with HRT

Disease	Reduced number of cases per 1000 women using HRT for 5 years	Reduced number of cases per 1000 women using HRT for 10 years
Colorectal cancer	1 reduced case with use of oestrogen alone or combined HRT in users <59 years old	2 reduced cases with use of oestrogen alone or combined HRT in users <59 years old
	3 reduced cases in users between 60 and 69 years old	5–6 reduced cases in users between 60 and 69 years
Fractured neck of femur	1 reduced case with use of oestrogen alone or combined HRT in users <59 years old	1 reduced case with use of oestrogen alone or combined HRT in users <59 years old
	2–3 reduced cases in users between 60 and 69 years	5 reduced cases in users between 60 and 69 years

* This is according to the Million Women Study. According to the WHI, there are 4 extra cases of breast cancer per 1000 women taking combined HRT for 5 years and no extra cases in women on oestrogen alone.

CHAPTER 7:
PAEDIATRICS

CHAPTER 7:
PAEDIATRICS

The NSF for children, young people and maternity services

This National Service Framework (NSF) was published in September 2004 and sets out national standards for children's health and social care. It also aims to improve the health of women in pregnancy and early motherhood. It is envisaged that the standards set out will be met by 2014.

Standards

Part 1

Standard 1: Promoting health and well-being, identifying needs and intervening early

The health and well-being of all children and young people is promoted and delivered through a co-ordinated programme of action, including prevention and early intervention wherever possible, to ensure long-term gain, led by the NHS in partnership with local authorities.

Standard 2: Supporting parenting

Parents or carers are enabled to receive the information, services and support which will help them to care for their children and equip them with the skills they need to ensure that their children have optimum life chances and are healthy and safe.

Standard 3: Child, young person and family-centred services

Children and young people and families receive high-quality services which are co-ordinated around their individual and family needs and take account of their views.

Standard 4: Growing up into adulthood

All young people have access to age-appropriate services which are responsive to their specific needs as they grow into adulthood.

Standard 5: Safeguarding and promoting the welfare of children and young people

All agencies work to prevent children from coming to harm and to promote their welfare, provide them with the services they require to address their identified needs and safeguard children who are being or who are likely to be harmed. Primary Care Trusts (PCTs) have an obligation to ensure that all families in their area who are not registered with a GP are offered registration.

Part 2

Standard 6: Children and young people who are ill

All children and young people who are ill, or are thought to be ill or injured will have timely access to appropriate advice and to effective services which address their health, social, educational and emotional needs throughout the period of their illness.

Standard 7: Children and young people in hospital

Children and young people receive high-quality, evidence-based hospital care, developed through clinical governance and delivered in appropriate settings.

Standard 8: Disabled children and young people and those with complex health needs

Children and young people who are disabled or who have complex health needs receive co-ordinated, high-quality child and family-centred services which are based on assessed needs, which promote social inclusion and, where possible, which enable them and their families to live ordinary lives.

Standard 9: The mental health and psychological well-being of children and young people

All children and young people, from birth to their eighteenth birthday, who have mental health problems and disorders have access to timely, integrated, high-quality multidisciplinary mental health services to ensure effective assessment, treatment and support, for them and their families.

Standard 10: Medicines for children and young people

Children, young people, their parents or carers, and healthcare professionals in all settings make decisions about medicines based on sound information about risk and benefit. They have access to safe and effective medicines that are prescribed on the basis of the best available evidence.

Part 3

Standard 11: Maternity services

Women have easy access to supportive, high-quality maternity services, designed around their individual needs and those of their babies.

Every child matters

Inadequacies in children's social care have been highlighted in the past few years by high profile cases such as that of Victoria Climbié, a little girl who died of neglect and abuse, despite being known to health and social services. This and other similar cases prompted the Government to draw up a green paper entitled '*Every Child Matters*', published in September 2003, which set out plans to reform services for young people. Its aim is to strengthen child protection services for the most vulnerable children and, rather ambitiously, to ensure that all young people have 'the best opportunities in life'. The delivery strategy '*Every Child Matters: Next Steps*' was published in 2004 and will be co-ordinated with the children's NSF delivery strategy.

There are four main areas of focus:

✓ Early intervention in child protection is emphasised and children known to more than one agency will have a key-worker. Teachers, social workers and other professionals will work together in multidisciplinary teams based in schools and children's centres. These children's centres will offer integrated early years education and support for families.

✓ Accountability and integration. Local Authority education and social services will be amalgamated. Every council will have to set up a **children's trust** by 2006, bringing together health, education and social services. The trusts will include community and acute health services, such as community paediatrics, teenage pregnancy co-ordinators, child and adolescent mental health services and speech and language therapy. PCTs will be expected to work closely with these children's trusts, and will delegate responsibility for commissioning relevant services. Senior managers will be involved with child protection issues. A director of children's services will head the trusts and be accountable for education and social services within the local authority.

✓ Supporting parents and carers. GPs and schools will take on responsibility for helping to provide parents and families with more support and advice, including parenting classes. There are plans for a 24-h helpline for parents.

✓ Workforce reform. There will be more input from nurses, midwives and health visitors in child protection. There will be standardised training for all staff working with children.

There is an independent child commissioner whose job it is to protect the welfare of young people, monitor Government policy and investigate serious child protection failures.

Implications for primary care

On average, pre-school children visit their GP six times a year, compared to two to three times a year for school-age children. GPs are therefore well placed to help with the implementation of some of the targets set out in the NSF.

Child Health Promotion Programme

This replaces the Child Health Surveillance Programme. Its aim is to move away from a limited number of routine developmental checks to a more holistic assessment of the needs of the child and family. There is much emphasis on health promotion and on the need for early intervention to address identified needs.

Safeguarding children

GPs are expected to keep detailed records of all consultations (there should ideally be a single set of medical records from which all health professionals work), particularly when concerns have been raised about the child's welfare.

The term 'safeguarding' is now used instead of child protection. It is recommended that all practice personnel involved in the care of children should have regular training and updates in this area.

A guidance document entitled 'What to do if you're Worried a Child is being Abused' has been published by the Department of Health. In cases of suspected abuse, the child and family should be referred to Social Services. Social Services are obliged to acknowledge the referral in writing within one working day.

Prescribing for children

The new children's British National Formulary (BNF) has now been distributed to all GPs and will be reviewed annually. Concordance is often a particular problem in children and adolescents and regular medication reviews are important. Certain practical points should be remembered, such as trying to prescribe medicines which can be taken on a once-daily or twice-daily basis; ie out of school hours. It is sometimes necessary to provide two prescriptions, one for school and one for home.

Looking after teenagers

The specific health needs of young people are often neglected by primary care as it is believed that adolescents are on the whole a healthy group who rarely present to their GP (BMJ 2005; **330**: 465). Improving services to allow young people to engage with their health will result in both short-term and long-term population health gains (BMJ 2005; **330**: 901).

Practices are expected to be 'teenage-friendly' and to provide 'targeted and sensitive' care to help address issues such as teenage pregnancy, smoking, substance misuse, sexually transmitted infections (STIs) and mental health problems. There should be posters up in surgeries detailing their confidentiality policy. The importance of access to confidential contraceptive and sexual health advice services is particularly emphasised and all GPs should be familiar with the Fraser guidelines.

SUMMARY POINTS

✓ NSF sets standards for children's health

✓ Child protection services are improving

✓ Health promotion is vital

✓ Teenagers are often still neglected in primary care

USEFUL WEBSITES

www.doh.gov.uk – Department of Health

www.bnfc.org/bnfc – Children's BNF

Childhood vaccinations

MMR vaccination

The percentage of children aged 2 years in England who had received the measles, mumps and rubella (MMR) vaccine rose from 80% in 2003–4 to 81% in 2004–5. This is the first year-on-year increase since 1995–6.

In some areas, herd immunity is being jeopardised and there is concern that the incidence of measles is increasing as a result of the reduced uptake of the vaccination. Certainly, outbreaks of measles have occurred in London, where MMR uptake rates are among the worst in the country.

An ecological analysis of national data on hospital admissions found no increase in Crohn's disease associated with the introduction of the MMR vaccination programme, providing strong evidence against the hypothesis that MMR vaccine increases the risk of Crohn's disease (*BMJ* 2005; **330**: 1120–1121).

A Japanese research study has provided the strongest proof yet that the MMR vaccination does not cause autism, by showing that rates of autism in Japan continued to rise even after the triple vaccine was withdrawn (*J Child Psychol Psychiatry* 2005; **46(6)**: 572–579).

Four independent bodies have reviewed the evidence: the CSM, the Joint Committee on Vaccination and Immunisation, the Medical Research Council (MRC) expert group and the Committee on the Safety of Medicines (CSM) Working Party on MMR Vaccine. They have all agreed that there is no evidence to suggest that the MMR has any long-term adverse effects. A recent Cochrane review (*Cochrane Library* 2005 issue 4) analysed 31 studies comparing the MMR vaccine to placebo, to no treatment and to the single antigen vaccines. The authors found evidence of short-term effects (eg febrile convulsions), but not of any long-term disability such as autism or inflammatory bowel disease. Andrew Wakefield, who was responsible for the initial scare, has now been thoroughly discredited, especially since allegations have been made of research misconduct and undeclared financial interests.

One qualitative study (*Br J Gen Pract* 2004; **54**: 520–525) based in five general practices in Leeds found that prior parental experience of autism was a powerful factor in influencing decisions about vaccination. Parents who had had close contact with autistic children tended to perceive the risks of acquiring measles, mumps or rubella as being less serious than the risk of the vaccine itself. The opposite was true for parents who had direct, personal knowledge of the impact of catching measles, mumps or rubella. In general, parents had a high level of trust in their GP and health visitor, although there were some concerns about lack of impartiality. Factors likely to support informed decision-making on MMR uptake included drop-in sessions at local nurseries or schools, written information (including case studies and pictures) and vaccination appointments with their GP. The study concluded that a personalised approach is preferable when imparting information about the MMR, taking into account the parent's level of understanding and past experiences.

Is there any place for single-antigen vaccines?

Some parents still have reservations about the MMR and would prefer to give their children single vaccines. When the single measles vaccine was used in the UK before 1988, there were regular epidemics of measles, with 10–20 deaths each year. There is no research evidence or experience of a regimen giving measles, mumps and rubella vaccines separately to preschool children. A link between the single vaccine and autism and bowel disease has never been investigated. It is not known what the optimum time interval between doses should be, or even if it provides adequate protection against the diseases. Children would need to have six injections instead of two. Because of the added inconvenience and distress that this would entail, there is a risk that parents would choose not to have their children immunised against all three diseases; this might result in decreased immunity rates and community outbreaks, which could be disastrous for vulnerable groups such as pregnant women and the immunocompromised.

All single measles and mumps vaccines available in the UK are unlicensed and therefore could be unreliable. Finally, no country in the world recommends the use of single measles, mumps and rubella vaccines as an alternative to the combined MMR vaccine.

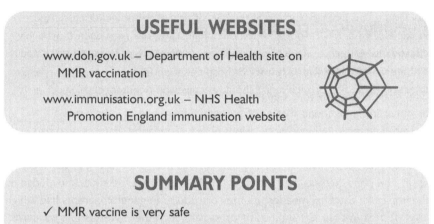

USEFUL WEBSITES

www.doh.gov.uk – Department of Health site on MMR vaccination

www.immunisation.org.uk – NHS Health Promotion England immunisation website

SUMMARY POINTS

✓ MMR vaccine is very safe

✓ Personalised approach best when imparting information about risk

✓ No evidence for single antigen vaccines

The 'five in one' vaccination

The pentavalent vaccine DTaP/Hib/IPV has now replaced the DtaP/HiB vaccine. It is still given at 2, 3 and 4 months of age. The main difference is that the polio vaccine was previously live and was administered orally while the new polio vaccine is inactivated and administered intramuscularly. Pertussis is now given in an acellular form instead of the previous whole virus vaccine; it will probably produce fewer side-effects such as fever and soreness at the injection site. The pentavalent vaccine is thiomersal free.

Meningitis C is still administered separately, also at 2, 3 and 4 months.

Chickenpox vaccination

All children aged between 12 and 18 months in the USA have been immunised against varicella zoster since 1995. This has led to a dramatic reduction in the incidence of chicken pox, with hospital admission rates dropping from 2.3 to 0.3 per 100,000 (*JAMA* 2005; **294**: 797–802). There is still debate about whether it should be introduced in the UK.

Pneumococcal conjugated vaccine

Children with chronic disease (eg respiratory disease, such as asthma, or diabetes) and those with a history of hospitalisation for lower respiratory chest infection (including bronchiolitis) should receive the pneumococcal vaccine.

CHAPTER 8:
CANCER

CHAPTER 8: CANCER

The NHS Cancer Plan

The NHS Cancer Plan was introduced in September 2000 and was the first comprehensive national cancer programme. Its aims were to:

- ✓ Save more lives.

- ✓ Ensure cancer patients receive correct professional support and care.

- ✓ Ensure patients receive the best available treatments.

- ✓ Tackle the inequalities in cancer healthcare.

A report called '*Tackling Cancer in England; Saving More Lives*' was published in 2004 (www.ngo.org.uk). It found that, overall, the incidence of cancer increased by 31% between 1971 and 2000 (perhaps due to better data collection). However, mortality fell by 12% between 1971 and 2002. Breast cancer mortality has decreased by 5–11% since screening was introduced in 1988.

How does the NHS Cancer Plan affect GPs?

All Primary Care Trusts (PCTs) have reviewed their cancer screening coverage and improved the uptake, especially by ethnic minorities and deprived patient groups. A national system of cancer networks has been set up which aims to plan cancer services to meet individual needs and co-ordinate cancer plan initiatives at a local level. A lead clinician for cancer should have been appointed for each PCT; this is a GP who has dedicated time to work for the cancer network and help to improve clinical standards. This GP also helps to improve communication across primary, secondary and tertiary services.

Cancer registers have also been established for each PCT and GPs contribute to these.

Cancer and the GMS Contract

Cancer is one of the diseases included in the GMS Contract.

To achieve maximum quality points, the following standards need to be met:

✓ The practice must have a register of all cancer patients diagnosed after April 2003.

✓ 90% of patients diagnosed after 1.4.03 should have had a review by the practice recorded within 6 months of the confirmed diagnosis. This should include an assessment of support needs and a review of co-ordination arrangements with secondary care.

What role should GPs play in cancer diagnosis and treatment?

GPs are very involved in managing patients with cancer. They are concerned with the comprehensive, co-ordinated and continuous care of individuals, families and, increasingly, populations. GPs have an important role in cancer and the Government's desire to improve cancer outcomes relies heavily on GPs playing their part.

Diagnosing cancer in primary care is often difficult. Many cancers present with common symptoms such as persistent cough or non-specific abdominal pain, yet few patients with such symptoms turn out to have cancer. Primary care clinicians need to be able to discriminate which patients within a relatively unselected population have a higher likelihood of malignant disease. The new NICE guidelines (see below) may go some way towards helping with diagnosis.

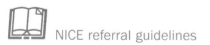 NICE referral guidelines

NICE published referral guidelines for suspected cancer in June 2005. These guidelines are directed at GPs, to help them to prioritise which patients require urgent referral and which investigations may be indicated. Cancers covered are lung cancer, upper gastrointestinal cancer, lower gastrointestinal cancer, breast cancer, gynaecological cancer, urological cancer, haematological cancer, skin cancer, head and neck cancer including thyroid cancer, brain and CNS cancer, bone cancer and sarcoma and cancer in children and young people.

Some of these referral guidelines are detailed in this chapter.

Upper GI cancer

Anyone with any of the following alarm symptoms and signs should be referred immediately, with the aim of being seen within 2 weeks: **chronic gastrointestinal bleeding; progressive, unintentional weight loss; progressive dysphagia; persistent vomiting; iron deficiency anaemia; epigastric mass or suspicious barium meal.**

Patients over 55 years old with persistent, unexplained (eg not related to NSAID ingestion) recent-onset dyspepsia alone should also be referred urgently even in the absence of 'alarm' signs and symptoms (this has changed since their 2004 guidance).

Patients with iron deficiency anaemia, persistent vomiting and weight loss should be considered for urgent endoscopy even if they do not have symptoms of dyspepsia.

Colorectal cancer

The following patients with bowel symptoms and signs should be referred urgently:

1. Patients aged 40 years and older, reporting rectal bleeding with a change of bowel habit towards looser stools and/or increased stool frequency persisting for 6 weeks or more.

2. Patients aged 60 years and older, with rectal bleeding persisting for 6 weeks or more without a change in bowel habit and without anal symptoms.

3. Patients aged 60 years and older, with a change in bowel habit to looser stools and/or more frequent stools persisting for 6 weeks or more without rectal bleeding.

4. Patients presenting with a right lower abdominal mass consistent with involvement of the large bowel, irrespective of age.

5. Patients presenting with a palpable rectal mass (intraluminal and not pelvic), irrespective of age.

6. Men of any age with unexplained iron deficiency anaemia and a haemoglobin of 11 g/100 ml or below.

7. Non-menstruating women with unexplained iron deficiency anaemia and a haemoglobin of 10 g/100 ml or below.

Risk factors

Patients with ulcerative colitis should have a plan for follow-up with a specialist – they are at increased risk of bowel cancer.

There is insufficient evidence to suggest that a positive family history of colorectal cancer can be used to decide whether to refer.

Investigations

In patients with equivocal symptoms, a full blood count may help in identifying the possibility of colorectal cancer by demonstrating iron deficiency anaemia.

In patients for whom the decision to refer has been made, no other examinations or investigations are indicated.

In patients with unexplained symptoms related to the lower gastrointestinal tract, a digital rectal examination should always be carried out, provided this is acceptable to the patient.

Lung cancer

All patients diagnosed with lung cancer should be offered information, both verbal and written, on all aspects of their diagnosis, treatment and care. This information should be tailored to the individual requirements of the patient, and audio and videotaped formats should also be considered.

Urgent referral for a chest radiograph should be offered when a patient presents with:

✓ haemoptysis,

or any of the following unexplained or **persistent** (that is, lasting more than 3 weeks) symptoms or signs:

✓ cough

✓ chest/shoulder pain

✓ dyspnoea

✓ weight loss

✓ chest signs

✓ hoarseness

✓ finger clubbing

✓ features suggestive of metastasis from a lung cancer (for example, in brain, bone, liver or skin)

✓ cervical/supraclavicular lymphadenopathy.

If a chest radiograph (CXR) or CT scan suggests lung cancer (including pleural effusion and slowly resolving consolidation), patients should be offered an urgent referral to a chest physician. If the CXR is normal but a high index of suspicion of lung cancer remains, the patient should still be referred urgently.

The following patients should be referred urgently to a chest physician without needing to wait for the results of a CXR:

✓ Persistent haemoptysis in smokers or ex-smokers >40 years old.

✓ Superior vena cava obstruction.

✓ Stridor.

USEFUL WEBSITES

www.doh.gov.uk

www.nice.org.uk

SUMMARY POINTS FOR CANCER

✓ New NICE referral guidelines for common cancers

✓ Lead clinician to be appointed for each PCT

✓ GPs have a crucial role in both cancer care and cancer screening

✓ Cancer is included in the GMS contract

Prostate cancer

Prostate cancer is now the most commonly diagnosed non-skin cancer in developed countries and over the last 20 years death rates from this disease have doubled. It is second only to lung cancer in terms of male cancer deaths. Men (with no family history of the disease) have a 1 in 12 lifetime risk (*BJU* 2000; **85**: 588–598), and its incidence is increasing. This appears to be a result of our aging population and the increasing use of prostate specific antigen (PSA) as a screening tool. Despite considerable advances in the ability to detect and treat prostate cancer, there have been no significant corresponding decreases in morbidity and mortality in the UK. In the USA, where prostate cancer screening with PSA testing widely occurs, prostate cancer mortality has been falling by around 3% per annum (although whether this is due to screening is debated).

Serum measurement of PSA (probably the most important tumour marker known to medicine) has led to a 'stage migration' where prostate cancer is increasingly detected at an earlier stage. Presently, however, we have no evidence that this will lead to a reduction in cancer-specific mortality. It has been estimated that anything from 29% (*J Natl Cancer Inst* 2002; **94**: 981–990) to 80% (*Can Med Assoc J* 1998; **159**: 1368–1372) of PSA-screen-detected cancers would, even without treatment, never become symptomatic and this represents a huge overdiagnosis of the disease. We should not forget, however, that prostate cancer is a heterogeneous disease with 30,000 men diagnosed with prostate cancer and 10,000 men dying from it in the UK in 2002.

What are the problems with measuring PSA levels in patients?

Poor specificity

PSA cannot distinguish between indolent slow growing tumours that pose no risk to health and those that are dangerous and aggressive in their behaviour.

PSA is organ specific and not tumour specific and therein lies the problem.

It can be raised due to:

- ✓ benign prostatic hyperplasia (BPH, proportional to the size of the gland)

- ✓ prostatitis

- ✓ urinary retention

✓ instrumentation of the urinary tract

✓ prostate biopsy

✓ ejaculation.

Prolonged recumbency and 5-alpha reductase inhibitors reduce PSA (the latter by half). Rectal examination has no effect. In order to increase its diagnostic accuracy, several concepts have been developed: age-adjusted upper limits, PSA density (concentration in relation to prostate volume), PSA velocity (change in concentration with time) and free/total PSA ratio (the lower the ratio the greater the likelihood of cancer). More recently interest has been focusing on various isoforms of proPSA (the precursor to PSA) and their ratio to PSA.

These concepts are of more use when deciding whether to subject patients to a second or even third round of biopsies or whether to simply monitor their PSA. Normal practice dictates that patients with a raised PSA (who have been appropriately counselled) undergo a prostate biopsy.

Around 25% of men with a PSA of 4–10 ng/ml will be found to have cancer, increasing to 35% with an immediate second round of biopsies. With PSA values of 10–20 ng/ml the pickup is over 60%.

It may be worthwhile repeating a raised PSA: a study of 972 men who were tested for PSA and had their PSA repeated 6 weeks later before the patient had a prostate biopsy (*JAMA* 2003; **289**: 2695–2700) found that the percentage of men whose high result returned to normal in a later test ranged from 44% to 55% (depending on the threshold). Of those who could be tested again after their level had dropped down to normal, 65–83% remained normal. This would spare men unnecessary biopsies.

The lower limit to trigger biopsy in the USA may change. Analysis of the Prostate Cancer Prevention Trial (PCPT) (*N Engl J Med* 2004; **350**: 2239–2246) has shown detection rates of around 25% for a PSA of 2.0–4.0 ng/ml (not dissimilar to that for 4.0–10 ng/ml). There are plans to change their present lower limit for biopsy to 2.0 ng/ml, which may well occur in the UK in the future.

Poor sensitivity

Unfortunately up to 20% of patients with prostate cancer do not have elevated levels of PSA and would therefore be overlooked (hence the importance of the digital rectal examination as an adjunct to any PSA test). A rather alarming study from the USA recently concluded that if their current PSA cut-off of 4.0 ng/ml is adhered to, then 82% of men under the age of 60 years who go on to develop prostate cancer would be missed, and a lower cut-off of 2.6 ng/ml was recommended by this paper (*N Engl J Med* 2003; **349**: 335–342).

Presently, PSA as a tool for population-based screening is being evaluated in large prospective randomised controlled trials in Europe and the USA. We are going to have to wait a further 5 years for the results to become available. Often with screening programmes, pressure is applied, supposedly by the public but more often from specific interest groups, to introduce screening and then, once established, further pressure is applied to reduce screening intervals and extend age ranges.

What is the optimal treatment for early prostate cancer?

Controversy exists about the treatment of apparently localised prostate cancer. This is partly because some prostate cancers develop slowly and may never cause problems in the patient's lifetime, hence any treatment of these is 'over treatment' (50% of men aged 80 have prostate cancer on autopsy studies, but only 4% die of it); however, other prostate cancers evolve rapidly and are fatal within a few years.

Radical treatment is generally not justified for patients with a PSA concentration over 20 ng/ml, as the tumour will often extend beyond the prostatic capsule and there may be micro-metastases or lymph node deposits. The grade of tumour and the life expectancy of the patient also influence the final decision. Patients with well-differentiated tumours may do well without treatment whereas those with poorly differentiated tumours usually do badly (*JAMA* 2005; **293**: 2095–2101). Most men have moderately well differentiated tumours and are likely to benefit from radical treatment only if they have a life expectancy of more than 10 years.

An American study examined the outcome over 14 years of men diagnosed with localised prostate cancer and found that for men with palpable but non-metastatic prostate cancer the mean time to death was 11.7 years (*BJU Int* 2000; **85**: 1063–1066). The authors of this study actually propose an upper age limit of 62 years for a screening programme when the intent is to cure. The difficulty obviously remains that some men in their 70s and 80s will present with metastatic bone disease and will leave us wondering whether this could have been prevented by screening.

Treatment for prostate cancer

There are three main treatments at present – radical prostatectomy, radical radiotherapy and brachytherapy. A fourth treatment, cryosurgery, which is freeze/thawing to destroy tissue, is currently gaining popularity. Radical treatment offers the potential for cure, but can also have serious side-effects, including post-operative pain and blood transfusion, hospitalisation, radiation proctitis and varying levels of impotence and to lesser extent incontinence. With active surveillance (previously known as watchful waiting), men have to live with the knowledge that they have an untreated cancer which may progress (and therefore has the potential, if not switched to a radical treatment in time, to be fatal).

In order to evaluate the most effective treatment for clinically localised prostate and, more importantly, to establish whether to introduce a screening programme for prostate cancer, the government is funding a £13 million phase III trial known as the ProtecT study (Prostate testing for Cancer and Treatment). Men aged 50–69 years with at least 10 years life expectancy are offered PSA testing after full counselling of the implications of a raised PSA. Those with PSA >3.0 ng/ml (but <20 ng/ml) undergo biopsies and if they are shown to have localised prostate cancer are offered a choice of radical prostatectomy, radical radiotherapy or active surveillance. Recruitment closes mid 2006 and the main endpoints will be survival at 5, 10 and 15 years, disease progression and treatment complications. Alongside ProtecT will run The Comparison Arm for ProtecT (CAP) Study to find out what happens to their unscreened peers. The results from both trials are eagerly awaited!

Until then we have to rely on studies such as the recent randomised controlled trial published by the Scandinavian Prostate Cancer Group (*N Engl J Med* 2005; **352**: 1977–1984). Nearly 700 men with organ-confined prostate cancer were randomised to either watchful waiting or radical prostatectomy. Over an 8.2-year median follow-up period 14.4% of patients on watchful waiting and 8.6% of patients who had undergone surgery died of prostate cancer. Radical prostatectomy reduced cancer-specific mortality by 44%. Furthermore, the difference in the rate of development of distant metastases of 25% versus 15% in favour of surgery was taken to show that ongoing follow-up of the trial will further show the clear benefit of radical prostatectomy (median survival once distant metastases are present is 2–3 years). The benefit in terms of disease-specific mortality and overall mortality was small but statistically significant. It is questioned as to whether these results are applicable to screen-detected cancers (whose natural history is more favourable) as this trial used clinically detected cancers. Twenty men would require radical prostatectomy to prevent one death over 10 years and this number needed to treat (NNT) may be as high as 40 for screen-detected cancers (*BJU* 2005; **96**: 954–956). This seems small benefit.

Can we prevent prostate cancer?

The largest urological study to date involving over 18,000 men – the Prostate Cancer Prevention Trial – has been published (*N Engl J Med* 2003; **349**: 213–222). This investigated whether the use of finasteride – a 5-alpha reductase inhibitor that prevents the conversion of testosterone to dihydrotestosterone, which is the active androgen in the prostate – would prevent prostate cancer. The trial was stopped prematurely at 7 years when finasteride did indeed achieve a 24.8% reduction in the prevalence of prostate cancer compared with placebo (period prevalence of 24.4% with placebo compared to 18.4% when taking finasteride). This is the first time that medical intervention has been shown to conclusively reduce the prevalence of prostate cancer to a clinically meaningful extent.

There were, however, a few concerns. There was a very high rate of cancer detection in both groups more in keeping with autopsy study rates than previous screening studies. Hence, due to the study design in which everyone was subjected to a biopsy, a large number of 'insignificant' cancers were found. Also, there was, worryingly, a greater proportion of poorly differentiated cancers amongst the finasteride group. Could it be that the price you pay for reducing the number of cancers overall is the development of a greater proportion of higher grade more aggressive and hence worse prognosis cancers? We don't know the answer.

Should prostate cancer be screened for?

Media publicity and a heightened public awareness of prostate cancer have increased the profile of PSA screening. The question of whether screening should be implemented is still hotly debated. At present, PSA testing for prostate cancer does not fulfil all of Wilson's criteria for screening (See 'Screening' on page 214).

The National Screening Committee has advised against screening as:

- ✓ Many subclinical cases would be detected.

- ✓ Excess anxiety would result.

- ✓ In many cases there would be no change in the overall outcome.

- ✓ The PSA level cannot predict whether the cancer is indolent or aggressive.

- ✓ PSA has a poor specificity.

- ✓ There is still a lack of consensus regarding treatment for early disease.

✓ Physical harm of prostate biopsies.

✓ Some cancers detected would never present clinically.

There are also strong arguments towards introducing a screening programme including:

✓ Men's autonomy.

✓ PSA is a cheap and readily available test.

✓ Screening may possibly be beneficial (lack of evidence of effectiveness does not prove ineffectiveness).

✓ May lead to detection of early, potentially curable cancers.

One report found that PSA screening causes overdiagnosis rates of prostate cancer in about 29% of white men; many men whose cancers were diagnosed through PSA screening would likely have died of a disease other than prostate cancer (*J Natl Cancer Int* 2002; **94**: 981–990). In addition, this report stated that most of the prostate cancers (85%) detected via PSA testing in recent years would have presented clinically.

Two American studies have shown that screening men for prostate cancer has no impact on death rates from the disease. One study examined the outcomes of more than 1000 men with prostate cancer. Half of the patients had been screened using PSA test alone or in combination with a rectal examination. The other half had not been screened at all. The patients were followed up for 4–9 years and the conclusion was that PSA screening did not improve survival in men under 70 years (*J Clin Epidemiol* 2002; **55**: 603). The other compared prostate-cancer-specific mortality over an 11-year period in Connecticut and Seattle. Seattle's intensive PSA screening (over 5-fold that of Connecticut) and increased treatment (6-fold increase in radical prostatectomy and 2.5-fold increase in radiotherapy) made no difference to disease-specific survival from prostate cancer (*BMJ* 2002; **325**: 740–744). This again demonstrated the burden of overdiagnosis.

To illustrate what PSA screening would mean I can find no better explanation than the following quote from Professor Neal (one of the key instigators of ProtecT): 'The balance of proof must be high to justify exposing men older than 50 years to a process where, of 1 million men, about 110,000 with raised PSAs will face anxiety over possible cancer, about 90,000 will undergo biopsy, and 20,000 will be diagnosed with cancer. If 10,000 of these men underwent surgery, about ten would die of the operation, 300 will develop severe urinary incontinence, and even in the best hands 4000 will become impotent. The number of men whose prostate cancer would have impinged on their lives is unknown.'

What are the NHS prostate cancer screening policy recommendations?

These were implemented in July 2001 and recommend that when a patient requests a PSA test, he should be given full information on the advantages and disadvantages of testing. The National Electronic Library for Health has produced patient information leaflets available online. These vary from a one-page summary to a detailed five-page leaflet, so can supposedly be 'tailored' to the patient's level of interest.

Under the policy, the NHS will not be inviting men for PSA testing and does not expect GPs to raise the subject of PSA testing with their asymptomatic patients. However, the Government policy states that 'any man considering a PSA test will be given detailed information to enable him to make an informed choice about whether to proceed with a test or not'. This therefore implies that asymptomatic men may have the test if they want, so there is now ambiguity about whether screening is supported and confusion about what this policy means in everyday practice.

An assumption has been made that most men will not want to be tested once they are informed of the uncertainties. However, in the feasibility study for the ProtecT trial, around 90% of men given detailed information about the implications of PSA testing and the lack of evidence about treatment consented to a test!

The proof of the ability of PSA testing to reduce the disease-specific mortality of prostate cancer will be provided by randomised controlled trials, which are currently underway in both USA and Europe. Unfortunately it will be many years before these results are available and, in the interim, doctors must act on the information that is currently available in the best interests of their patients. Patients must be informed of the pros and cons of PSA testing and also the implications of a positive result before having a PSA test performed.

SUMMARY POINTS FOR PROSTATE CANCER

✓ Incidence of prostate cancer is rising

✓ Screening may occur in future (ProtecT trial now running)

✓ Controversy exists over optimum treatment for early prostate cancer

✓ Finasteride has been shown to reduce the risk of developing prostate cancer

Screening for bowel cancer

Bowel cancer is very common; there are more than 30,000 new cases of colorectal cancer each year in the UK and the average 5-year survival rate is 40%. Risk increases with increasing age.

Now that the UK Colorectal Cancer Screening Pilot has been completed, a national screening programme is due to be rolled out in April 2006.

The UK colorectal cancer screening pilot was set up to examine the feasibility of screening for colorectal cancer with faecal occult blood test screening (FOBT). In this pilot study, which involved 480,000 people in Tayside, Grampian, Fife and the West Midlands, uptake rates were approximately 60% (although rates were much lower in the Muslim population at 30%; men generally and people in deprived areas were less likely to accept screening).

Despite its relatively poor sensitivity (60–70%) and specificity, it was estimated that FOBT would save 1200 people per year from dying of colon cancer in England (*BMJ* 2004; **329**: 137). For every 1000 patients screened, 2 cases of colon cancer might be detected, and another 3–4 of polyps. The cost of screening was about £5900 per life year saved.

It has therefore been agreed that colorectal cancer screening for people aged 60–69 will be rolled out from April 2006, using FOBT; patients over the age of 70 will be screened on request. Potential problems include cost, availability of endoscopy and training issues. One in 50 people screened is likely to test positive and will need to be referred for colonoscopy. This would NOT fall under the 2-week wait.

Flexible sigmoidoscopy is an alternative method of screening. In a trial in the USA, 84% of people aged 55–74 took up the invitation for screening, out of a total of 77,465 (*J Natl Cancer Inst* 2005; **97**: 989–997). Twenty-three per cent had at least one polyp and the eventual cancer detection rate was 3 per 1000 patients screened. However, a recent American study has found that this approach would miss two-thirds of important lesions (*N Engl J Med* 2005; **352**: 2061).

A study has shown that, surprisingly, women are less likely to attend for a flexible sigmoidoscopy than men (*J Med Screening* 2005; **12**: 20). This is mainly because women think that the investigation is going to be embarrassing or humiliating. This is despite the fact that women are more likely to perform FOB testing at home compared to men.

A study to determine the impact of the UK Colorectal Cancer Screening Pilot on primary care workload was recently published (*Br J Gen Pract* 2005; **55**: 20–25). Forty per cent of GPs thought that a national colorectal screening programme would substantially impact on workload. This is after most practice staff said that they spent less than 2% of their time during the screening period on Pilot-related activities. Whether or not adequate resources and training will accompany the screening programme remains to be seen.

Advantages of FOBT

✓ Can be done at home

✓ Acceptable

✓ Non-invasive.

Disadvantages of FOBT

✓ Has to be repeated every 2 years

✓ Poor sensitivity (60–70%)

✓ Poor specificity (5% false positives)

✓ Results in large numbers of colonoscopies; the NHS does not currently have the resources to cope with this.

Mammography

Mammography is currently offered to all women between the ages of 50 and 70 in the UK. There is much controversy about whether routine mammography has helped to increase survival from breast cancer, and if so by how much. Some experts claim that increased survival is due to better treatments and earlier diagnosis; although the majority view is that mammography has also played a part.

Mortality rates from breast cancer are falling, both in women who undergo mammography and in women who don't.

A 20-year follow-up study of breast screening and its effect on mortality concluded that breast screening can reduce mortality rates in women aged between 40 and 74 by 23% (and by 48% in women aged 40–49) (*Lancet* 2003; **361**: 1405–1410). It warned that 'until formal methods are developed for partitioning mortality changes by attribution to screening, treatment and other factors, the percentage reduction in mortality from screening remains unknown and incalculable'.

Mammography may be effective in women from the age of 40 according to the first 10-year estimates from the UK Age trial (*Br J Cancer* 2005; **92**: 949–954). This is looking specifically at the impact of mammography in 53,000 women aged between 40 and 50 who are receiving annual screening. Detection of invasive breast cancers has been 8% higher in the screening group than in controls. Sensitivity of first screen has been 74% and 54% at subsequent screens. Detection of invasive breast cancers has been 0.09% at the first and subsequent screens. Uptake has been 68–70%.

A recent article attempted to use a particular statistical model (the Markov model) to estimate benefits and harms of biennial screening mammography for women aged 40, 50, 60 and 70 years (*BMJ* 2005; **330**: 936–938).

They concluded that:

- ✓ For every 1000 women screened over 10 years, 167–251 receive an abnormal result (depending on age).

- ✓ 56–64 of these women undergo at least one biopsy.

- ✓ 9–26 have an invasive cancer detected by screening.

- ✓ 3–6 have ductal carcinoma in situ (DCIS) detected by screening.

- ✓ More cases of invasive breast cancer and of DCIS are diagnosed in screened women. For example, at the age of 50, for every 1000 women who have 5 biennial screens, 8 extra cases of invasive breast cancer will be detected, and 5 cases of DCIS.

- ✓ Overall, there are projected to be about 0.5, 2, 3 and 2 fewer deaths from breast cancer over 10 years per 1000 women aged 40, 50, 60 and 70 respectively who choose to be screened compared with women who decline screening.

Problems with mammography

Up to 20% of breast cancers detected are DCIS. These localised cancers have an uncertain natural history, and early detection may lead to unnecessary mastectomies, particularly in older women with co-existing morbidity whose life expectancy is limited anyway (this is similar to the prostate cancer treatment argument).

Mammography would be expected to increase the incidence of breast cancer in women in the target age range for screening, with a reduction in the incidence of cancer in older women who have already undergone screening (on the premise that many cancers that would have developed in older women would be detected earlier with screening). This is not necessarily the case however; analysing breast cancer incidence rates in Norway and Sweden it has been found that cancer incidence in women aged between 50 and 69 increased substantially after the implementation of screening, without any commensurate decline in breast cancer incidence in older women (*BMJ* 2004; **328**: E301–E302).

✓ Mammography is about 90% sensitive in women over 50 who are not on hormone replacement therapy (HRT), so 10% of cancers are missed. It is probably less sensitive in women on HRT.

✓ It is not particularly specific: 10% of women will have an abnormal mammogram, but of these only about 5% will truly have breast cancer. Clearly, false positives lead to a great deal of anxiety.

✓ It is an uncomfortable and potentially embarrassing procedure.

✓ A Cochrane review re-analysed all the existing trial data supporting mammography in 2001 and concluded that there was no evidence to prove a survival benefit of mass screening for breast cancer. The methodological quality of the major trials evaluating mammography was criticised in this review. This was preceded by another review which came to the same conclusions (*Lancet* 2000; **355**: 129–134).

Arguments for mammography

✓ Experts from the World Health Organization (WHO) have concluded that mammography helps to cut death rates from breast cancer by about a third and have directly refuted the reviews quoted above. These experts re-examined the original studies and found that they were indeed reliable (*BMJ* 2002; **324**: 695).

✓ Of the 21% fall in breast cancer mortality since 1991, 6% is estimated as being due to screening, and 15% due to better treatment (*BMJ* 2000; **321**: 665).

✓ A large Swedish meta-analysis showed a significant reduction in mortality in screened compared to non-screened women (*Lancet* 2002; **359**: 909).

✓ There may be fewer mastectomies and more breast-conserving surgery in screened women who are diagnosed earlier (*BMJ* 2002; **325**: 418).

Cervical cancer

Cervical screening

All women aged between 25 and 49 years should be screened every 3 years and women aged between 50 and 64 years should be screened every 5 years.

Effectiveness of the cervical screening programme (*Lancet* 2004; **364**: 249)

✓ Researchers examined trends in mortality before 1988 when the UK national screening programme was launched, in order to try to predict what future trends in cervical cancer mortality would have been without screening.

✓ Cervical cancer mortality in women under 35 rose threefold between 1967 and 1987, so that by 1988 the UK incidence of cervical cancer in this age group was one of the highest in the world.

✓ Since the introduction of screening in 1988, these rising mortality rates have been reversed; the authors of the study claim that were it not for screening, 1 in 65 women born after 1950 would have died from cervical cancer and that the screening programme saves up to 5000 lives per year.

✓ Cost per life-year saved is approximately £36,000.

NICE guidance on liquid based cytology (LBC) 2003

With LBC, samples are collected in the usual way using a spatula or brush. The head of the device is rinsed or broken off into a vial of preservative fluid so that the majority of cervical cells are retained. Samples are then transported to the lab.

NICE has recommended that LBC should replace Pap smears. This is mainly because of the lower rate of inadequate smears when LBC is used; UK pilot studies have shown a statistically significant decrease in the number of inadequate samples from 9.1% with Pap slides to 1.6% with LBC. Overall sensitivity with LBC was improved by 12% compared with the Pap smear, but specificities are similar.

Screening

A screening procedure is one that is applied to a population to select people at risk of an unfavourable health outcome for further investigation, monitoring or advice and treatment. Informed choice with regard to screening is essential because although screening programmes may benefit populations, not all participants will benefit and some will even be harmed by participation (*BMJ* 2002; **325**: 78–80).

What is informed choice?

Informed choice has two core characteristics – it should be based on relevant, good-quality information and the resulting choice should reflect the decision-maker's values. The GMC has produced guidance on the information that should be provided to people offered screening.

What are Wilson's criteria for screening?

These well-established criteria should ideally be met before implementing a screening programme. They are important to know and can be applied to other screening programmes as well as to different types of cancer. There are, however, very few conditions for which all the criteria can be met.

They state that:

- ✓ The condition should be common and important.
- ✓ There must be a latent period or early symptomatic stage during which effective treatment is possible.
- ✓ There must be acceptable and available treatment for the disease.
- ✓ The untreated natural history of the disease must be known.
- ✓ The screening tests must be acceptable, cost-effective, safe and reliable.
- ✓ The screening test should be highly sensitive and specific.
- ✓ The screening should be continuous (not just a 'one off' test).

What are the ethics of screening?

The four main principles of ethics should be applied here (they are very useful to know for the viva exam!):

✓ Beneficence (do good)

✓ Non-maleficence (do no harm)

✓ Autonomy

✓ Justice.

Beneficence

The benefit of screening must outweigh any potential harm to an individual.

Non-maleficence

Personal costs include problems with false-positive results, which can lead to distress and possible unnecessary treatment. False-negatives can also occur, as no test is 100% sensitive, which can then lead to false reassurance by both patients and doctors. This may even dissuade patients from returning for future screening tests.

Misinterpretation of results can lead to a false sense of security, for example patients with normal cholesterol or normal blood pressure may continue to smoke. There are also the costs to society, the actual costs of equipment, services, treatment, etc and also the time taken off work for people to attend for the screening test and the treatment.

Finally, there are psychological costs involved. One article showed that false-positive results in screening tests can have undesirable effects (*J Public Health Med* 2001; **23**: 292–300). Women who had been given the 'all clear' after having had abnormal mammography results 3 years previously remained significantly more anxious than those who had normal results. This was actually sufficient to deter 15% of them from attending for mammography the next time round.

Autonomy

Some people have different health beliefs and cultures and object to being screened. This needs to be appreciated when considering individual autonomy.

Justice

Implementing screening tests may mean that funds are diverted away from other services, for example cancer treatments. The correct allocation of limited resources is very important, especially in the current climate.

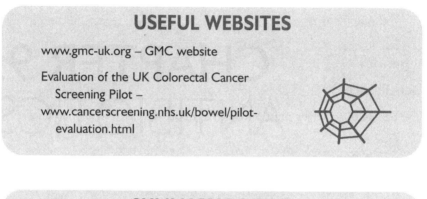

USEFUL WEBSITES

www.gmc-uk.org – GMC website

Evaluation of the UK Colorectal Cancer
  Screening Pilot –
www.cancerscreening.nhs.uk/bowel/pilot-
  evaluation.html

SUMMARY POINTS

✓ Colorectal cancer screening is due to start soon

✓ Mammography may be effective from 40 years

✓ Cervical screening programme is extremely successful

CHAPTER 9:
ANTIBIOTICS

CHAPTER 9:
ANTIBIOTICS

The debate of antibiotic prescribing and resistance continues to remain at the forefront of much of the research that takes place within primary care. Many of the studies summarised here are pivotal in changing prescribing patterns within the GP population in the UK. Some of the studies included are intended to stimulate thought about your own prescribing methods and to highlight much of the uncertainty that still remains.

Antibiotic resistance

Antimicrobial resistance describes the ability of a microorganism to resist the growth-suppressing or microbicidal effects of particular antimicrobial agents. This ability can reflect a naturally occurring property of an organism (eg having a thick cell wall) or might develop through alteration of the organism's genes. In some cases, genes conferring resistance to a particular antimicrobial can be transferred between different strains of microorganisms, the recipient organisms thus becoming resistant.

Emergence of antimicrobial resistance in infectious organisms at a population level is dependent on the survival and further spread of organisms with antimicrobial resistant properties. The extensive use of antimicrobial agents probably helps this process along, by eliminating sensitive microorganisms, which in turn allows the resistant ones a greater opportunity to spread.

Antibiotic misuse is common and studies have suggested up to 70% of treatment courses are unnecessary or inappropriate. Treatment with antibiotics is often unnecessarily prolonged, inappropriate or given at the wrong time. One major factor affecting the prescribing behaviour of GPs is the expectations of their patients.

The Standing Medical Advisory Committee (SMAC) Report

In July 1997, the Chief Medical Officer asked the SMAC to examine the issue of antimicrobial resistance in relation to medical prescribing.

Recommendations for treatment were as follows:

✓ No prescribing of antibiotics for simple coughs and colds.

✓ No prescribing of antibiotics for viral sore throats.

✓ Limit prescribing for uncomplicated cystitis to 3 days in otherwise fit women.

✓ Limit prescribing of antibiotic agents over the telephone to exceptional cases.

USEFUL WEBSITES

http://www.advisorybodies.doh.gov.uk/smac1.htm – full report available

www.hpa.org.uk/infections/topics_az/antimicrobial_resistance/ menu.htm – General information and the latest antimicrobial resistance data from the Health Protection Agency

---

SUMMARY POINTS FOR ANTIBIOTIC RESISTANCE

✓ 80% of antibiotic use is in the community

✓ 50% of community use is for respiratory tract infections, 15% for urinary tract infections

✓ Considerable local and regional variations exist in the levels of community prescribing

Antibiotic prescribing in general practice and hospital admissions for peritonsillar abscess, mastoiditis, and rheumatic fever in children: time trend analysis (*BMJ* 2005; **331**: 328–329)

This study focused on the possible association between reduced prescribing and an increased incidence of rare complications of bacterial infection, in particular peritonsillar abscess, mastoiditis and rheumatic fever in children during 1993–2003.

Data were extracted for children aged ≤15 years. The most substantial decline in the prescribing rate of antibiotics by GPs (34%) occurred before 1999. After 1999, prescribing by GPs seemed to level off, falling only by a further 3%.

✓ From 1993 to 2002, hospital admissions for peritonsillar abscess and rheumatic fever did not increase.

✓ Hospital admission rates for mastoiditis and simple mastoidectomy increased by 19% (from 6.9/100,000 to 8.2/100,000).

✓ This rise was attributable predominantly to an increase in admissions among children aged ≤4 years.

✓ However, the data from the general practice research database did not confirm an increase in mastoiditis or referral for mastoidectomy.

The authors commented that over the past decade antibiotic use resulting from GP prescribing of antibiotics to children has halved, and this reduction has not been associated with an increase in admission to hospital for peritonsillar abscess or rheumatic fever. The decline in use was due initially to a substantial reduction in prescribing by GPs. After 1997 the proportion of prescriptions taken to a pharmacist also declined, possibly indicating that the 'delayed prescribing' policy was being adopted.

The reduction in general practice events could reflect the fact that children with suspected serious complications such as mastoiditis are increasingly being taken direct to hospital. The best estimate is that a minimum of 2500 children need to be treated with an antibiotic to prevent one case of mastoiditis.

Urinary tract infections

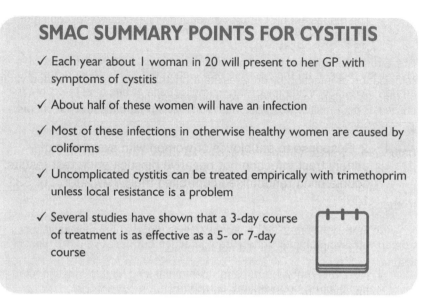

SMAC SUMMARY POINTS FOR CYSTITIS

✓ Each year about 1 woman in 20 will present to her GP with symptoms of cystitis

✓ About half of these women will have an infection

✓ Most of these infections in otherwise healthy women are caused by coliforms

✓ Uncomplicated cystitis can be treated empirically with trimethoprim unless local resistance is a problem

✓ Several studies have shown that a 3-day course of treatment is as effective as a 5- or 7-day course

1. Presence of bacteriuria caused by trimethoprim resistant bacteria in patients prescribed antibiotics: multilevel model with practice and individual patient data (*BMJ* 2004; **328:** 1279–1301)

This study attempted to ascertain evidence of a relation between antibiotic resistance and prescribing by GPs by analysis of prescribing at both practice and individual-patient level. They also wanted to test the hypothesis that, in comparison with practice-level data, analysis of individual patient data would reveal a much stronger association between antibiotic exposure and resistance.

✓ Repeated cross-sectional study in 1995 and 1996.

✓ The main outcome measure was resistance to trimethoprim in bacteria isolated from urine samples at the practice and individual level simultaneously in a multilevel model.

✓ Practices showed considerable variation in both the prevalence of trimethoprim resistance (26–50% of bacteria isolated) and trimethoprim prescribing (67–357 prescriptions per 100 practice patients).

✓ The association with trimethoprim resistance was strongest for people recently exposed to trimethoprim.

✓ The results support efforts to reduce unnecessary prescribing of antibiotics in the community.

These results show that recent antibiotic exposure increases the risk of colonisation or infection by drug-resistant bacteria and show the added value of analysis of data for individual patient prescribing.

2. Response to antibiotics of women with symptoms of urinary tract infection but negative dipstick urine test results: double blind randomised controlled trial (*BMJ* 2005 16; **331**: 143)

The objective was to assess the effectiveness of antibiotic treatment for women with symptoms of urinary tract infection but negative urine dipstick testing.

✓ Prospective, double-blind, placebo RCT.

✓ Participants: 59 women aged 16–50 years presenting with a history of dysuria and frequency in whom a dipstick test of midstream urine was negative for both nitrites and leukocytes.

✓ Intervention: trimethoprim for 3 days or placebo.

✓ Results showed the median time for resolution of dysuria was 3 days for trimethoprim compared with 5 days for placebo.

✓ The median duration of constitutional symptoms (feverishness, shivers) was reduced by 4 days.

✓ The authors concluded that although a negative dipstick test for leukocytes and nitrites accurately predicted absence of infection when standard microbiological definitions were used (negative predictive value 92%), it did not predict response to antibiotic treatment. Three days' treatment with trimethoprim significantly reduced dysuria in women whose urine dipstick test was negative.

These results support the practice of empirical antibiotic use guided by symptoms. Balancing the competing interests of symptom relief and the minimisation of antibiotic use remains a dilemma.

The findings are ultimately opposed to current policy that actively attempts to reduce antibiotic prescribing in the UK. The trial could be criticised for its small sample size and for lack of mid-stream urine results.

Sore throat

When should we use antibiotics?

Antibiotics have been used in the past to:

- ✓ Reduce the severity or shorten the duration of symptoms.

- ✓ Reduce the risk of complications: suppurative (quinsy, otitis media, sinusitis) and non-suppurative (rheumatic fever, nephritis).

- ✓ Satisfy non-clinical purposes, eg perceived patient demand.

We now have evidence to help us select those patients who probably have a bacterial infection and may benefit from penicillin. The Centor criteria:

patients with high fever, purulent tonsillitis, cervical lymphadenopathy and no concurrent cough are more likely to have bacterial infection

These Centor criteria have been criticised as cervical adenitis and lack of cough were found to be the most sensitive markers for bacterial infection (*Br J Gen Pract* 2005; **55**: 615–619).

SMAC SUMMARY POINTS FOR SORE THROAT

- ✓ Most are viral and can be left to run their course without resort to antibiotics

- ✓ Recurrence and relapse may be more common in those who have had early treatment with antibiotics

- ✓ Those who receive antibiotics are more likely to return for treatment for future attacks and are more likely to believe in the efficacy of antibiotics

- ✓ Qualitative studies in the UK over the past decade have found that doctors overestimate patients' expectations for antibiotics

1. Penicillin for acute sore throat: randomised double blind trial of 7 days vs 3 days treatment or placebo in adults (*BMJ* 2000; **320**: 150–154)

Patients with sore throats for less than 7 days and with three of the four 'Centor' criteria were included:

- ✓ fever
- ✓ no cough
- ✓ tonsillar exudate
- ✓ swollen, tender, anterior cervical nodes.

The trial showed that penicillin V for 7 days resulted in:

- ✓ Two days' shorter duration of symptoms
- ✓ Reduced incidence of complications (quinsy)

Supports the use of penicillin V in patients with three of the four Centor criteria.

2. Why do general practitioners prescribe antibiotics for sore throat? Grounded theory interview study (*BMJ* 2003; **326**: 138)

This study explored GPs' reasons for prescribing antibiotics for sore throat and the factors that influenced their decision making.

- ✓ Face-to-face, open ended interviews.
- ✓ Results showed GPs are uncertain which patients will benefit from antibiotics but prescribe for sicker patients and for patients from socioeconomically deprived backgrounds.
- ✓ They are also more likely to prescribe in pressured clinical contexts.
- ✓ GPs are uncertain who benefits most from antibiotics for sore throat and are particularly concerned about complications.

The authors concluded that GPs have reduced prescribing for sore throat in response to research and policy but further interventions to reduce prescribing would need to improve identification of patients at risk of complications and be workable in busy clinical situations.

Otitis media

Acute otitis media (AOM) is a common condition with a high morbidity and low mortality.

In the UK, about 30% of children aged under 3 years have acute otitis media each year. It is the most common reason for children to be prescribed antibiotics by their GPs.

Factors predisposing to poor outcome include: multiple previous episodes, bottle feeding, history of ear infections in parents or siblings and use of a pacifier (dummy).

In 80% of children the condition resolves without antibiotic treatment in about 3 days.

Antibiotics give limited benefits and most children can be treated without them.

Benefits of withholding antibiotics include reduced cost, reduced side-effects and reduced antibiotic resistance.

SMAC SUMMARY POINTS FOR AOM

✓ Reviews on AOM suggest that the benefit of routine antimicrobial use is unproved or modest. Although a proportion of children do benefit, it is difficult to predict which ones

✓ Countries with lower rates of antibiotic prescribing for AOM show no increase in the number of complications compared with those where a prescription is usual

✓ Even if antibiotics are prescribed, there is debate about the appropriate length of treatment: if antibiotics are prescribed, the course should be limited to 3 days

Suggested evidence-based management

Explain that:

- ✓ Most patients get better within 24 h without antibiotics.

- ✓ Most cases are due to viruses.

- ✓ Offer a prescription of antibiotic if symptoms are not starting to settle after 72 h.

- ✓ Consider giving information leaflets.

- ✓ Consider deferred prescription of antibiotic, only to be used if the child is no better after 24–48 h.

- ✓ Consider an antibiotic at the outset if the child is unduly ill, toxic or has a high fever.

Pragmatic randomised controlled trial of two prescribing strategies for childhood acute otitis media (*BMJ* 2001; **322**: 336–342)

This clinically useful, large RCT study looked at the rationale behind delayed prescriptions in general practice.

- ✓ Children were randomised to receive immediate treatment or delayed treatment with support from standardised advice sheets.

- ✓ Outcome measures were symptom resolution, absence from school or nursery and paracetamol consumption.

- ✓ On average, symptoms resolved after 3 days.

- ✓ Children in the immediately prescribed antibiotic group had a shorter duration of illness (–1.1 days), fewer disturbed nights (–0.72 days) and slightly less paracetamol consumption.

- ✓ 24% of the children given delayed prescriptions used antibiotics and 77% of parents were very satisfied.

- ✓ Fewer parents in the delayed group believed in the effectiveness of antibiotics and in the need to see the doctor for future episodes.

In conclusion, immediate antibiotic prescription provided symptomatic benefit mainly after the first 24 h, when symptoms were already resolving. For children who are not very unwell systemically, a wait-and-see approach seems feasible and acceptable to parents and should substantially reduce the use of antibiotics for acute otitis media.

A recent Cochrane review of eight trials found that antibiotics led to no reduction in pain at 24 h but a 30% relative reduction at 2–7 days (*The Cochrane Library*, Issue 2, 2005). As 80% of patients will have resolved spontaneously in this time, absolute benefits are small (only 7%).

Respiratory tract infections

1. Information leaflet and antibiotic prescribing strategies for acute lower respiratory tract infection: a randomized controlled trial (*JAMA* 2005; **293:** 3029–3035)

This recent study by Little looked at prescribing strategies in general practice for antibiotics.

- ✓ RCT involving 807 patients over 5 years (1998–2003).

- ✓ Patients were assigned to six groups by a factorial design: leaflet or no leaflet and one of three antibiotic groups (immediate antibiotics, no offer of antibiotics, and delayed antibiotics).

- ✓ An information leaflet had no effect on the main outcomes.

- ✓ Compared with no antibiotics, other strategies did not alter cough duration or other primary outcomes.

- ✓ The authors concluded that a 'no offer' or a delayed offer of antibiotics for acute uncomplicated lower respiratory tract infection (LRTI) is acceptable, associated with little difference in symptom resolution and is likely to considerably reduce antibiotic use and beliefs in the effectiveness of antibiotics.

2. Variations in antibiotic prescribing and consultation rates for acute respiratory infection in UK general practices 1995–2000 (*Br J Gen Pract* 2005; **55:** 603–608)

This investigated whether general practices that issue fewer antibiotic prescriptions to patients presenting with acute respiratory infections had lower consultation rates for these conditions.

- ✓ The results found that the practices which prescribe antibiotics to a smaller proportion of patients presenting with acute respiratory infections have lower consultation rates for these conditions.

- ✓ Practices that succeed, over time, in reducing antibiotic prescribing also experience reductions in consultation rates for these conditions.

3. Do delayed prescriptions reduce antibiotic use in respiratory tract infections? (*Br J Gen Pract* 2003; **53**: 871–877)

✓ Analysis showed the relative risk in the randomised trials for lower antibiotic usage when a delayed prescription was given ranged from 0.54 for the common cold to 0.25 for otitis media.

✓ Consistent reduction in antibiotic use for the common cold, acute cough and otitis media.

✓ The duration of delay for prescriptions ranged widely, from 1 to 7 days.

✓ Patients are less likely to think antibiotics will work if given a delayed script.

✓ Patients may be less satisfied if given a delayed script as opposed to asking them to return to collect it.

✓ They concluded that there was a consistent reduction in antibiotic usage in the five controlled trials and that delayed prescription is an effective means of reducing antibiotic usage for acute respiratory infections.

4. Patients' responses to delayed antibiotic prescription for acute upper respiratory tract infections (*Br J Gen Pract* 2003; **53**: 845–850)

GPs frequently issue such prescriptions simply because they believe that the patient expects it. The aim of this study was to establish the proportion of recipients who claim to consume their delayed antibiotic prescriptions and to elicit factors associated with patients' decisions.

✓ 87% were confident about taking the decision about whether to use their antibiotics.

✓ 92% would choose to receive a delayed prescription again.

✓ Patients with fever or sinus pain were more likely to use antibiotics.

✓ It appears most patients are confident in making the decision.

SMAC SUMMARY POINTS FOR DELAYED ANTIBIOTICS

✓ GPs constantly try to reduce antibiotic prescribing

✓ Rates of serious infections are not likely to rise with a reduction in antibiotic prescribing

✓ Education leaflets do not provide additional benefits

Acute conjunctivitis

Chloramphenicol treatment for acute infective conjunctivitis in children in primary care: a randomised double-blind placebo-controlled trial (*Lancet* 2005; **366**: 37–43)

This recent pivotal study looked at the very frequent complaint of childhood conjunctivitis.

✓ One in eight schoolchildren has an episode of acute infective conjunctivitis every year.

✓ Standard clinical practice is to prescribe a topical antibiotic, although the evidence to support this practice is limited.

✓ This was a double-blinded RCT to compare the effectiveness of chloramphenicol eye drops with that of placebo in children within primary care.

✓ Eye swabs were taken for bacterial and viral analysis.

✓ Clinical cure by day 7 occurred in 83% of children treated with placebo compared with 86% of those given chloramphenicol.

✓ The study showed no statistically significant benefit of antibiotics compared to placebo.

However, the likely impact of these findings on prescribing patterns is uncertain. Parental anxiety and pressure for treatment, particularly in an environment where schools will not allow attendance until treatment has been given, continue to promote prescribing.

CHAPTER 10: CLINICAL GOVERNANCE

CHAPTER 10: CLINICAL GOVERNANCE

Definition: 'A system through which NHS organisations are accountable for continuously improving the quality of their services and safeguarding high standards of care and creating an environment in which excellence in clinical care will flourish.'

What are the components of clinical quality?

✓ Professional performance (technical quality)

✓ Resource use (efficiency)

✓ Risk management (risk of injury or illness associated with the service)

✓ Patient satisfaction.

What can we do to improve?

✓ Audit

✓ Review complaints

✓ Critical incident reporting

✓ Routine surveillance.

Why is it needed?

✓ GP quality is too variable

✓ Patients have a right to expect improved consistency in access to, and quality of, primary care services

✓ Patients need to be assured that their treatment is up to date and effective and is provided by 'up to date' doctors.

In reality

- ✓ Doctors must take part in audit
- ✓ Leadership skills must be developed within clinical teams
- ✓ Evidence-based medicine must be practised
- ✓ Good practice must be disseminated
- ✓ Risk management procedures must be in place
- ✓ Adverse events must be detected and investigated
- ✓ Lessons learnt must be applied to clinical practice
- ✓ Poor performance must be recognised early and tackled promptly.

How does it work in Primary Care Trusts (PCTs)?

- ✓ Each PCT has nominated a senior professional to lead on clinical standards and professional development
- ✓ Each practice must have a named clinical governance lead, responsible for liaising with the rest of the primary healthcare team (PHCT) and with the PCT
- ✓ Information on quality (audits) may become public and identifiable as lay members of the PCT may demand it and other doctors may want it.

Conclusions

- ✓ The advent of clinical governance is a watershed in the history of general practice
- ✓ Each GP is to be responsible for providing high-quality care, auditing care, auditing their own standards and those of their colleagues in the PCT
- ✓ Clinical governance is a powerful tool for improving quality of care in general practice
- ✓ Clinical governance is hence a means of maintaining quality assurance and accountability to the public
- ✓ It may be our last chance for self-regulation.

SANDWELL & WEST BIRMINGHAM NHS TR.

	Qty	Sales Order		10930001 F

Ship To:
SANDWELL & WEST BIRMINGHAM
SANDWELL DISTRICT HOSPITA
LYDON
WEST BROMWICH
WEST MIDLANDS
B71 4HJ

Bill To: 10930000
SANDWELL & WEST BIRMINGHA
FINANCE DEPT, BROOKFIELD
DUDLEY ROAD
BIRMINGHAM
WEST MIDLANDS
B18 7QH

Routing

Sorting
Y07A06X
Covering — BXXXX
Despatch

ISBN	Qty	Sales Order	
9781904627722	1	F 9125037	1

Cust P/O List
23.50 GBP

Customer P/O No
78103

Fund:

Title: Hot Topics for MRCGP and General
Practitioners

Format: Paperback
Author: Newson, Louise
Publisher: PasTest
Volume:
Edition: 4Rev Ed   Year: 2006

Order Specific Instructions

National Institute for Clinical Excellence (NICE)

NICE gives guidance by:

✓ Appraisal of evidence

✓ Development and dissemination of audit methods

✓ Development and dissemination of guidelines

✓ Effectiveness bulletins.

The Healthcare Commission (previously The Commission for Health Improvement – CHI)

✓ Looks at clinical governance at PCT level

✓ Visits a random selection of practices

✓ Provides a collaborative approach with poorly performing PCTs

✓ Can report underperforming health bodies to the Health Secretary

✓ Tells us whether we are following guidance by:

- Provider and service reviews

- Performance indicators

- Troubleshooting problem areas.

Papers

The following papers, although not essential to the exam, would provide you with a more in-depth understanding of the practical problems facing general practice in the current political climate. A few key points are summarised for those who, understandably, would find it tedious to venture further.

1. What's the evidence that NICE guidance has been implemented? Results from a national evaluation using time series analysis, audit of patients' notes, and interviews (*BMJ* 2004; **329**: 999)

This study assessed the extent and pattern of implementation of guidance issued by NICE.

- ✓ Interrupted time series analysis, review of case notes, survey, and interviews.

- ✓ All primary care prescribing, hospital pharmacies; a random sample of 20 acute trusts, 17 mental health trusts and 21 primary care trusts; and senior clinicians and managers from five acute trusts.

- ✓ Outcome was measured by rates of prescribing and use of procedures and medical devices relative to evidence-based guidance.

- ✓ 6308 usable patient audit forms were returned.

- ✓ Implementation of NICE guidance varied by trust and by topic.

- ✓ Prescribing of some taxanes for cancer and orlistat for obesity significantly increased in line with guidance.

- ✓ Prescribing of drugs for Alzheimer's disease and prophylactic extraction of wisdom teeth showed trends consistent with, but not obviously a consequence of, the guidance. Prescribing practice often did not accord with the details of the guidance.

- ✓ No change was apparent in the use of hearing aids, hip prostheses, implantable cardioverter defibrillators, laparoscopic hernia repair, and laparoscopic colorectal cancer surgery after NICE guidance had been issued.

The authors conclude that implementation of NICE guidance has been variable. Guidance seems more likely to be adopted when there is strong professional support, a stable and convincing evidence base and no increased or unfunded costs, in organisations that have established good systems for tracking guidance implementation and where the professionals involved are not isolated.

There is evidence that NICE guidance has been less influential in surgical procedures and use of medical devices. NICE guidance seems to have had an uneven impact on the uptake of evidence-based medicine.

2. Education and debate: challenges for the National Institute for Clinical Excellence (*BMJ* 2004; **329**: 227–229)

In summary:

- ✓ NICE has focused on evaluating new technologies rather than existing ones.

- ✓ This approach is creating inflationary pressure that the NHS cannot afford.

- ✓ Even with recent large increases in NHS expenditure, acute funding difficulties continue to emerge.

- ✓ Rationing involves depriving patients of care from which they may benefit and which they wish to have; this is inescapably the business of NICE.

- ✓ Rationing is the inevitable corollary of prioritisation and NICE must fully inform rationing in the NHS.

- ✓ The issue is not whether but how to ration.

- ✓ The criteria determining access to care depend on the health goals society is seeking to achieve. Are we solely interested in efficient use of resources – maximising health from a given budget? Or does society seek efficiency and equity and, if so, is it prepared to sacrifice some efficiency to achieve equity goals?

- ✓ Adoption of new technologies by NHS clinicians should be informed by costs as well as effectiveness.

- ✓ NICE appraisal should focus not only on service enhancement but also on withdrawal of existing ineffective or inefficient therapies.

- ✓ Giving NICE a real budget to fund its recommendations would encourage it to examine the effect of its decisions on the whole NHS.

3. Education and debate: making clinical governance work
(*BMJ* 2004; **329**: 679–681)

This article looked at the apparent failure of clinical governance implementation in the NHS. The author argues the true ethos and benefit has been lost through excessive bureaucracy. In summary:

- ✓ The current focus on quality and safety means most doctors have negative views about clinical governance.

- ✓ However, clinical governance has the power to improve NHS performance.

- ✓ The Government's past preoccupation with delivery and top-down performance management has undermined its developmental potential.

- ✓ As a bottom-up mechanism, it was intended to inspire and enthuse and create a no-blame learning environment characterised by excellent leadership, highly valued staff, and active partnership between staff and patients.

- ✓ The clinical governance arrangements established meet the formal requirements of central bodies such as the **Healthcare Commission**.

- ✓ The failure to take account of variations in clinical work has two main effects on clinical governance:

    1. It is removed from the day to day concerns of clinical staff.

    2. By divorcing issues of risk and safety from the specifics of providing care to a nominated patient group, the prevailing model encourages clinicians to view clinical governance as a management-driven exercise that has exploded their paperwork to the detriment of patient care.

If clinical governance is going to work, its developmental focus needs to be strengthened. This requires implementation of a model which recognises clinicians' central role in the design, provision and improvement of care. The model must also be structured to change how clinical work is conceived, performed and organised.

The self governance of clinical performance and organisation by multidisciplinary teams require structures and practices that will encourage multidisciplinary teams to engage in conversations that are focused on the detailed composition of care for specific conditions. Such conversations would deal with questions such as:

✓ Are we doing the right things?

✓ Are we doing things right?

✓ Are we keeping up with new developments and what are we doing to extend our capacity to undertake clinical work in these areas?

At the practice level, it requires the development and implementation of integrated care pathways for high volume case types. Clinicians are at the core of clinical work and should also be at the heart of clinical governance.

4. Clinical governance in primary care: participating in clinical governance (*BMJ* 2000; **321**: 737–740)

This paper emphasised the need for clinicians to find information that will improve their own practice and aid learning in the primary care team as a whole. Such work is likely to go a long way towards fulfilling the GMC's requirements for revalidation.

The NeLH (The National Electronic Library for Health) will eventually help to improve access to information in the practice. In one English region only 20% of GPs had access to bibliographic databases in their surgeries and 17% to the World Wide Web.

PCTs will need to invest in adequate information technology hardware, software and training. In England and Wales, Prodigy software is available free of charge on 85% of computer systems; it can offer advice during consultations on what to do in over 150 conditions commonly seen in primary care.

The MIQUEST project is one of the national facilitating projects within the NHS information management and technology strategy.

It aims to help practices standardise their data entry and provides software to help with data extraction, including data required for national performance indicators.

5. Using clinical evidence (*BMJ* 2001; **322**: 503–504)

Points raised:

- ✓ Most health carers want to base their practice on evidence and feel that this will improve patient care.

- ✓ It has proved too difficult, alongside the competing demands of clinical practice, to implement the original ideas that each health professional should: formulate questions themselves; search, appraise and summarise the literature; and apply the evidence to patients.

- ✓ Over 90% of British GPs believe that learning evidence-handling skills is not a priority, and even when resources are available, doctors rarely search for evidence.

- ✓ However, 72% often use evidence-based summaries generated by others, which can be accessed by busy clinicians in seconds.

- ✓ The NHS provides many of its clinicians with one of those sources – *Clinical Evidence*. This is a compendium of summaries of the best available evidence about what works and what doesn't work in healthcare.

Clinical Evidence presents the evidence, but does not tell doctors or patients what to do because evidence is only part of making a clinical decision. Clinical expertise to evaluate each patient's circumstances and personal preferences is also important. Even the best available evidence may need adapting for individual patients. Thus a valid, relevant and accessible source of detailed clinical evidence is a necessary, but not sufficient, precursor of innovation to achieve evidence-based healthcare. Additional professional, educational and operational support for clinical innovation will probably accelerate the use of clinical evidence.

Clinical Evidence will provide access to evidence in the way the *British National Formulary* provides access to prescribing information, and earn as welcome a place in the consulting room.

CHAPTER 11:
REVALIDATION

CHAPTER 11: REVALIDATION

Self-regulation

Self-regulation is whereby a profession determines its own training, qualifications and codes of ethics and behaviour.

This has been threatened by recent events such as:

- ✓ Loss of confidence by public.

- ✓ Perception that the profession closes ranks to protect its own interests.

- ✓ Demands for greater transparency and accountability.

- ✓ Being undermined by a less deferential and better-informed public.

Arguments for self-regulation

- ✓ A doctor's performance can only be adequately judged by someone doing the same job.

- ✓ Self-regulation engenders self-respect and motivation to perform well.

- ✓ Self-regulation helps to maintain professionalism and gives doctors a direct interest in maintaining standards.

- ✓ Without self-regulation, doctors would cease to be members of a profession.

Organisation of self-regulation

- ✓ Mechanism of revalidation to be supportive, not punitive, and largely by peer review, not examination.

- ✓ Poor performance must be recognised early, and intervention must be sympathetic but decisive.

- ✓ Support/retraining for any underperforming doctor must be available.

- ✓ Removal from the Register to be used as last resort, only for those beyond help.

✓ Overall, self-regulation must be robust and open to scrutiny, to avoid accusations of professional protectionism.

✓ The 'Council for the Regulation of Healthcare Professionals' is an overarching body. Its function is to regulate all the health professions and will exercise independent oversight of the General Medical Council (GMC), although it is not in itself a regulatory body. Its principal concern is the interest of patients and it can question a GMC judgement if it feels the latter has been too lenient.

Latest arrangements for revalidation

✓ Revalidation will mean that all doctors will have to demonstrate regularly to the GMC that they are up to date and fit to practise medicine.

✓ It will also enable doctors to identify and correct any weaknesses they may have.

✓ Doctors who are successful will be granted a licence to practise.

✓ Doctors who choose not to participate in revalidation will be able to stay on the register without the entitlement to exercise the privileges currently associated with registration.

✓ If concerns are raised about a doctor's 'Fitness to Practise' during the revalidation process, they will be referred to the GMC's Fitness to Practise procedures.

✓ There will be three stages to revalidation: collection of information; 5- or 7-year assessment; GMC decision.

1. Collecting information and yearly appraisal

Doctors have to collect evidence, which will be considered against the seven headings set out in the GMC guidance 'Good Medical Practice':

1. Good clinical care

2. Maintaining good medical practice

3. Teaching and training, appraising and assessing

4. Relationships with patients

5. Working with colleagues

6. Probity

7. Health.

These headings have also been used to structure the annual appraisal.

Sufficient information for headings 1–5 should be available from the documentation summaries of the appraisals. Doctors are asked to sign declarations about their health and their probity (including past criminal convictions).

During the appraisal, evidence being collected should help to identify any shortcomings in the doctor's performance, which can be addressed. However, if there is serious concern that the doctor poses a risk to themselves or to patients they should be referred to the GMC immediately.

2. Five- or seven-year assessment?

✓ The situation as far as formal revalidation is concerned remains unclear following the publication of the fifth Shipman report and the current re-think that is occurring as a result.

✓ Applies to NHS and non-NHS doctors.

✓ It is an assessment to check that the doctor is fit to practise.

✓ Both doctors and members of the public will be used to help consider the evidence.

✓ It is expected that the majority of doctors will be recommended for revalidation.

✓ If necessary the GMC will invoke the Fitness to Practise procedures.

✓ May or may not include a test of clinical competence. If it does include a test then perhaps the time frame will be extended to 7 years to account for this additional requirement.

3. The GMC decision

✓ The third and final stage is the GMC decision.

✓ It is expected that most doctors will be granted a licence to practise.

✓ However, if, as a result of the revalidation process, a doctor is considered under the Fitness to Practise procedures, then a number of outcomes are possible, including conditions placed on their practice or suspension.

✓ Effective action will be taken to protect patients.

1. Editorial: Where next with revalidation? (*BMJ* 2005; **330**: 1458–1459)

✓ Self-regulation should survive, but revalidation must offer education as well as performance review.

✓ Revalidation is necessary and must be comprehensive.

✓ In his article, Irvine espouses the view that doctors are personally responsible for their own ability to provide good care and that they share in the collective responsibility for their colleagues. In this context, revalidation is an essential expression of professionalism and a means of establishing accountability to patients and the public.

✓ Unfortunately, despite both professional obligation and patients' expectations, the performance of doctors declines over time.

✓ A recent systematic review found that, compared with their younger colleagues, older doctors and those in practice for more years had less factual knowledge; they were less likely to adhere to standards for diagnosis, screening, prevention and treatment; and their patients had poorer outcomes.

✓ Revalidation should focus on performance in practice.

2. Education and debate: GMC and the future of revalidation, time for radical reform (*BMJ* 2005; **330**: 1385–1387)

This editorial discusses the impact of recent publicised events on the changes to our regulatory authorities. The authors have also tabulated the key changes that have taken place over the last decade in a succinct format.

The authors argue that public and political faith in the professions and their regulators is lower than ever before, and resulted in part from authoritative criticism in several public inquiries, most notably Bristol and Shipman.

Recent legal reforms created a new Council for Healthcare Regulatory Excellence to oversee the regulators. The Council has the power to refer regulators' decisions on fitness to practise that it regards as unduly lenient to the High Court for review.

In the wake of the Shipman Inquiry, the Department of Health (DoH) has established not one but two reviews to explore the further reform of medical regulation and non-medical professional regulation.

The author argues that changes to professional regulation show an incremental and piecemeal approach to reform, lacking in any sense of wider vision or strategic direction. They are a collection of essentially reactive and short-term solutions to immediate problems, often made in the context of a single professional group without reference to other professions.

Such a fundamental reassessment is now long overdue. The authors believe it should consider four main issues:

1. Harmonising professional regulation

2. Defining the scope of professional practice explicitly

3. Maintaining actual professional competence more rigorously

4. Improving the governance and accountability of the health professions.

The author puts forward a notion that we should regulate not the professional title but the acts that a practitioner can undertake. This means defining an explicit scope of practice for each professional group, founded on a common set of regulated acts (diagnosis, investigation, prescribing, surgical intervention, etc). Each group would have a detailed definition of the acts practitioners can undertake and hence of the competencies they must have. When new professional groups arise, the question of whether they should be regulated is easily dealt with by examining whether they undertake regulated acts. When a group wishes to extend its role, it is again more straightforward to define the regulated acts this entails and, consequently, the competencies that need to be acquired and assessed. The question of who regulates a group becomes less important when the scope of practice is explicitly defined in a common terminology and when common standards for managing competence and fitness to practise are in place.

The author states that a genuine test of clinical competence needs to be in place for all healthcare professionals and that it should be based around the explicit scope of practice and defined competencies. It should be sufficiently flexible to respond to organisational context and evidence of performance, so that professionals who give cause for concern are monitored more intensively. Fundamentally, it must be a real examination of actual clinical competence and not some substitute or dubious proxy.

Professional regulatory reform in the UK: a brief chronology

1995   GMC publishes first edition of *Good Medical Practice*, setting out the duties of a doctor.

Medical (Professional Performance) Act 1995 passed, giving the GMC new powers to deal with problems of poor performance.

1999   Health Act gives the Government powers to reform professional regulation through Statutory Section 60 orders without the need to pass new primary legislation.

Department of Health publishes *Supporting Doctors, Protecting Patients*, which calls for a fundamental review of professional self-regulation and sets out 17 principles.

2000   Medical Act (Amendment) Order approved allowing GMC powers to make interim suspensions, restricting restoration of erased doctors, and widening membership of conduct committees.

NHS Plan outlines the intent to establish a UK Council for Health Care Regulators for the formal coordination of professional regulatory bodies.

2001   Bristol Royal Infirmary inquiry recommends creation of a body to oversee professional self-regulation and Department of Health publishes proposals for such reforms in *Modernising Regulation in the Health Professions*.

2002   Passage of the NHS Reform and Health Professions Act 2002, creating the Council for the Regulation of Health Professions (CHRP) with statutory powers of oversight over the regulators.

Medical Act (Amendment) Order 2002 approved enabling introduction of revalidation, new fitness to practise procedures, and changes in governance for GMC.

2003   CHRP (now known as the Council for Healthcare Regulatory Excellence) established and starts its first work programme, including performance reviews of all regulatory bodies and development of guidance on how to use its statutory powers.

2004   First referrals of some regulators' fitness to practise decisions to the Appeal Court on grounds of undue leniency. Appeal Court changes some decisions and refers some others back to the regulatory body for reconsideration.

Introduction of regulation for operating department practitioners by the Health Professions Council.

GMC introduces new fitness to practise rules with a single complaints process to replace separate conduct, performance and health proceedings.

Shipman Inquiry fifth report extensively reviews both old and new GMC fitness to practice procedures and criticises GMC for failing to protect the public and instead acting in the interests of doctors.

2005   Department of Health suspends adoption of new revalidation procedures by GMC and announces two reviews of medical and non-medical professional regulation.

3. Editorial: after Shipman: reforming the GMC – again
(*Br J Gen Pract* 2005; **55**: 83–84)

This editorial by the Editor of the *British Journal of General Practice* was published shortly after the Shipman Inquiry finally closed with a 1000 page report. In summary, the editorial argues, the Report poses fundamental questions for the whole medical profession.

It recommends:

- ✓ There should not be a majority of elected members on the Council.

- ✓ It should separate completely the investigative and adjudicative functions.

- ✓ It should have a much more stringent system for revalidation than the one that was due to be introduced at the time of the Report.

- ✓ Recommends adding a test of knowledge.

- ✓ To allow for a more demanding procedure it recommends intervals of every 7 rather than every 5 years.

- ✓ It should have direct accountability to Parliament as well as intermittent formal reviews of its procedures.

However, the Report advocates that the GMC should continue to be responsible for the fitness to practice procedures and hence supports self-regulation. Within days of its publication, it was announced that plans for revalidation were being postponed to take into account the Inquiry's recommendations.

Dame Janet Smith is to be congratulated for her willingness to adopt the unfashionable line in favour of self-regulation and for spelling out the reasons:

- ✓ That the GMC has changed its procedures in the light of some problems that have already emerged from the high profile scandals of the last few years.

- ✓ That it would be difficult to create an entirely new body to handle fitness to practice procedures.

- ✓ That it makes sense to keep the functions of licensing, revalidation and fitness to practice together as the responsibility of a single body.

- ✓ That primary care organisations (PCOs) should have more responsibility for handling local complaints, including being informed of all complaints made to practices.

The feeling of being continually under scrutiny could have a number of undesirable effects:

- ✓ Increase in defensive medicine, with patients suffering harm as a result.

- ✓ Likely to discourage the development of the 'no-blame culture' where we report all medical mishaps in the quest for continual, systematic improvement.

Protecting patients' interests must be the GMC's primary purpose, but doing that is the only way of restoring the reputation of the profession. We must hope that the distinction between human error and recurrent underperformance is one that the GMC can operate consistently and fairly in a way that will not open it, and by extension the rest of us, to the charge of excessive leniency.

4. GP experiences of partner and external peer appraisal: a qualitative study (Br J Gen Pract 2005; 55: 539–543)

Although UK guidance states that GP appraisal should be carried out by a practising GP, there is no indication if this should be carried out by a partner or an external colleague. In a previous study the most acceptable appraisers identified were externally appointed GPs from another practice or a peer partner from the same practice.

✓ The aim of the study was to explore GPs' perceptions of the advantages, disadvantages, threats and opportunities of being appraised by externally appointed GP colleagues and by their own partners.

✓ Sixty-six GPs agreed to take part in a study of partner and external peer-based appraisal.

✓ Six months later this group was followed up by questionnaire to determine views of the process.

✓ Appraisals were more likely to have occurred with an external appraiser.

✓ Issues raised in relation to having a practice or external appraiser included:

- lack of local/personal knowledge

- the impact of current practice dynamic, for example health, work efficiency or personality issues with or between partners

- the particular difficulties surrounding appraising more senior partners

- the resultant impact of these issues on evasion or collusion in the process.

✓ The issue of location was more important in the partner-appraised group, as the appraisal frequently took place in the appraiser's consulting room, creating feelings of a power imbalance.

✓ Protected time is essential for effective appraisal.

✓ This study reports the views of a small group of GPs who had volunteered to undergo appraisal, a less enthusiastic group of GPs might have different views of the appraisal process.

5. GP perceptions of appraisal: professional development, performance management, or both? (Br J Gen Pract 2005; 55: 544–545)

GPs' perceptions of the tension between the professional development and revalidation aspects of the current GP appraisal scheme were analysed.

✓ Three focus group interviews were held between April and June 2003:

1. GPs who had been appraised; selected to reflect a range of the total study population, namely those GPs who had been appraised in the pilot study.

2. GP tutors who had acted as appraisers.

3. The third consisted of the GP team who had planned and delivered the appraisal training.

✓ Focus group methodology was used to identify each group's responses, to generate qualitative data and to highlight needs.

✓ The results indicate that there is support for the professional development aspects of appraisal but the link with revalidation is problematic, thereby potentially undermining GP support for the scheme.

✓ Greater clarity about the precise nature of the linkage is required to avoid a process that fails to fully satisfy the requirements of either appraisal or revalidation.

✓ Some evidence indicates GP support for appraisal if it is focused on professional development, but they are apprehensive about a scheme that attempts to link professional development and assessment or revalidation.

✓ Appraisers and appraisees agreed that the process could be useful and that it encouraged them to reflect in a structured way on their professional role and development.

✓ Both groups highlighted perceived weaknesses in the scheme:

- they drew attention to the irrelevance of some of the exemplar material to the average GP

- the uncertainty as to whether resources would be made available to implement action plans

- the unsatisfactory nature of some aspects of the documentation

- the total emphasis on professional development and competence as opposed to the need for personal development as well.

✓ Concern was expressed at the lack of consistency and uniformity in the process, which could undermine its usefulness in revalidation.

✓ Study indicates that GPs are sceptical about the advisability of merging processes with conflicting aims.

✓ Appraisal can be a positive experience but further clarity about the process and linkages is needed.

National Clinical Assessment Authority (NCAA)

The NCAA offers a rapid performance assessment and support service for doctors:

✓ Will recommend monitoring, education, retraining, medical treatment or referral to the GMC

✓ Has special Health Authority status

✓ Health authority can refer doctors for advice and assessment

✓ Assessment carried out via practice visits

✓ Health authority will still be able to refer to GMC or deal with a doctor itself

✓ Assessors will be lay and medical

✓ GPs will be able to self-refer

✓ NHS pays for assessment

✓ GPs will have input

✓ Links with postgraduate deans and tutors

✓ Disciplinary action if GPs refuse to cooperate.

Practice and personal development plans (PPDPs)

Aims

✓ To combine personal self-directed learning with organisational development framework.

✓ To predispose to, enable and reinforce change, ie deliver information, rehearse behaviours and to provide reminders and feedback.

✓ To require learning portfolios for all members of the practice team (doctors, nurses, managers), taking into account the development needs both of individuals and the working unit.

✓ To involve the shift away from an individual performance to organisational performance as the measure of quality.

✓ To involve patients, which should ensure local responsiveness and prevent loss of personal care.

Ask yourself

✓ What do we need to do to improve our own practice?

✓ How have we identified what we need to do?

- Discussions

- Surveys

- Audits

- Significant event analysis

✓ Are these needs specific to our own practice, or do they reflect priorities in our Primary Care Trust (PCT) or the wider NHS?

✓ How are we going to address these needs?

✓ How will we judge our success?

✓ What do I need to improve the quality of care I provide? ('Reflection')

✓ How can I achieve these aims? ('Education')

✓ You choose your education on the basis of what you need to learn (Continuous professional development (CPD))

✓ A personal development plan (PDP) is part of the PPDP, as the team (practice) may require an individual to learn new skills in order to develop services.

Thus:

✓ There is much in common between Clinical Governance and PPDPs/PDPs.

✓ Education should help you maintain and improve the quality of your care.

The learning portfolio

Contains:

- ✓ All past significant sources and experiences of learning

- ✓ May include a description of your work and practice

- ✓ A summary of all your learning experiences

- ✓ A description of how you would like to develop professionally in the future

- ✓ Personal development plan would be at the heart of the learning portfolio

- ✓ Portfolio would act as a more long-term record of past experience and future aspirations.

Could include:

- ✓ workload logs

- ✓ case descriptions

- ✓ videos

- ✓ audits

- ✓ patient surveys

- ✓ research projects

- ✓ accounts of change or innovations

- ✓ reflective diaries on study and ongoing education.

CHAPTER 12:
THE FUTURE OF GENERAL PRACTICE

CHAPTER 12:
THE FUTURE OF GENERAL PRACTICE

Current problems

- ✓ Job satisfaction
- ✓ Morale
- ✓ Autonomy
- ✓ Workload
- ✓ Bureaucracy
- ✓ Recruitment
- ✓ Retention.

GP numbers threatened by

- ✓ More early retirement
- ✓ More part-time principals, women principals (career breaks)
- ✓ More doctors needed in secondary care
- ✓ Reduced immigration from outside the European Union (EU).

Possible solutions

✓ Increased medical school intake

✓ Increased resources for staff premises and technology

✓ Increased delegation to practice nurses (nurse practitioners)

✓ Limiting expansion of GPs' workload, especially from secondary to primary care

✓ Core contract changed to ensure GPs retain control of workload (variable, flexible, minimal, practice- rather than individual-based)

✓ Appropriate funding for care transferred from secondary to primary care

✓ Easier re-entry arrangements after a career break

✓ Flexible working arrangements

✓ Increased linking of practices through Primary Care Groups (PCGs), Primary Care Trusts (PCTs) and cooperatives

✓ Other health care professionals working in surgeries, eg pharmacists, physiotherapists, chiropractors, osteopaths, social workers, optometrists

✓ GPs employed by Community Trusts

✓ Initial triage by nurse practitioners – GP becomes specialist in family medicine (ie team leader) to be called upon only when needed

✓ Split contract – day and night elements.

Shaping tomorrow: issues facing general practice in the new millennium, GPC 2000

This was a discussion document issued by the General Practitioners Committee (GPC) of the British Medical Association (BMA); it gathered views from the profession, politicians and patients. Each subheading below is an area discussed, the salient points of which are summarised.

My doctor or any doctor quickly?

✓ Two apparent patient groups exist. The first group are essentially well and value easy access to healthcare with staff able to deal with their problem. The other comprises the chronically ill who place a high value on seeing their doctor.

✓ Divisions exist between GPs. Some feel that GPs overinvest in the notion of personal doctoring.

✓ However, the personal relationship is something that many patients do rate very highly.

✓ Many GPs see the personal relationship as central to what they do, others see it as a fading asset in a world of portfolio careers and part-time working.

✓ Advocates of personal lists point out that knowledge of the patient reduces expenditure (less investigation, etc).

✓ The demands of the well population must not be allowed to overshadow the demands and needs of the chronically unwell.

Independent contractor (IC) status versus salaried service: phoney war or real debate?

The arguments are for and against overlap, but essentially could be summed up as philosophical, clinical and financial – a heady enough mix to fuel any debate.

Pros to IC status:

✓ Allows GPs greater control of their jobs, ie ways of working, hours, staff, etc.

✓ Allows GPs to believe themselves to be other than 'mere employees of the State'.

✓ Allows us to be independent advocates for of our patients.

✓ Allows innovation, promotes entrepreneurial spirit, encourages change and efficiency.

✓ Leads to the development of vocational training, primary care teams, out-of-hours care and models of commissioning.

✓ It is a cheap service.

Cons:

- ✓ Young doctors don't want to buy into partnerships.

- ✓ Young doctors want a more flexible way of working.

- ✓ Researchers and academics complain of a data 'black hole' in general practice.

- ✓ A salaried system might stop GPs worrying about money and allow them to get on with doctoring.

- ✓ At its heart, independent contractor status has a lack of revalidation and supervision.

A job for life or portfolio careers

It isn't just changing patient expectations that will affect the shape of tomorrow's primary care – it's changing expectations among tomorrow's GPs. If young doctors do want part-time working, flexible careers, the chance to move practices every few years and the opportunity to mix general practice with other kinds of employment, then ultimately these desires need to be accommodated. There is a growing feminisation of the workforce, which raises issues around career breaks for motherhood and part-time working.

Clinical autonomy, does it have any place anymore?

In a world of NICE, NSF, guidelines and protocols, PRODIGY and clinical governance, does the concept of clinical autonomy still have any real meaning? Does this mean that GPs will lose the ability to mould care and treatment to individual patients? Many GPs take the view that guidelines and protocols are counsels of perfection, which are unobtainable under current resources. Yet doctors, rather than politicians, will be held to account, when it is not possible to deliver services to such standards.

Primary Care Trusts: working together or professional straitjacket?

Will Primary Care Trusts (PCTs) encourage GPs to work together in a more collective and cooperative way, or will they emerge as a new bureaucracy imposing a deadening uniformity and thereby extinguishing innovation and diversity?

Alongside new structures, a new public mood is emerging, which is demanding greater accountability from doctors, and a more transparent understanding of how they arrive at the judgements they do and what yardsticks are used in these decisions. In a narrow sense, it isn't immediately clear to whom PCTs will be accountable: Strategic Health Authorities? The NHS Executive? Ultimately to the Secretary of State, of course, but what will that mean for democracy on the ground?

In the wider sense of accountability, how will family doctors make it clear they want a genuine partnership with patients, and are they prepared to explain, and justify, what they do?

What do patients want?

It's an old joke, but it still raises a smile at every medical retirement party. When asked what was the best part of the job, the GP always says 'the patients'. Asked next what was the worst thing about the job, the GP always replies 'the patients'. So what should the relationship of the future be between GPs and patients? Everyone talks of partnership and the end of benign paternalism, and patient autonomy and shared care, sometimes; however, it is not hard to feel that the profession looks over its shoulder and rather wishes that 'doctor knows best' was still a politically correct option. If we are moving into a more honest and sharing relationship with patients, in which doctors are advisers and guides, there still seem few clear mechanisms for listening to what patients actually want, as opposed to doctors assuming they know what patients want.

If patients become clients, or even customers, does that make doctors into therapists and shopkeepers? And if it does, is that any bad thing? What do patients want? Patients' liaison groups, citizens' juries and patient advisory panels – this is the road we are going down. We need much better mechanisms to hear the voice of the patient. GPs can't carry on being paternalistic. The days of a submissive, subdued, semiliterate, lumpenproletariat, people who were underfed and had rotten lives of quiet desperation, are over.

Primary Care Trusts

Health authorities were abolished in 2002 and funding and commissioning of health services were devolved to PCOs (Primary Care Organisations) or Trusts. PCOs are overseen by the Strategic Health Authorities; SHAs might get involved if, for example, an acute trust (hospital) was in serious debt. Each PCT has a board, responsible for vision and values, strategies and planning. The board comprises a Professional Executive Committee (made up of five GPs, two or three nurses, one or two allied health professionals, the Director of Public Health, the Head of Social Services, the Director of Finance and the Chief Executive of the PCT, as well as pharmacists and dentists) and an executive committee.

The new GMS Contract

The new national contract was voted in, by a comfortable margin, in July 2003; a relief to the Government and the BMA after the rejection of the Consultant contract.

The new contract

This will be between the individual practice and the PCO, not the GP. There will be five different types of services, in which each practice will have to provide some or all of the following:

1. Essential services

These are mandatory and cover the provision of health care to everyone who is sick or 'believes themselves to be sick'; ie seeing patients in the traditional way. This covers emergency care and care for patients with chronic diseases.

2. Additional services

This comprises services such as child health surveillance, contraception, cervical screening, childhood immunisations, antenatal and postnatal care, ie services which most GPs routinely provide at present. Accordingly, under the new contract, most practices are expected to provide these services.

3. Directed enhanced services

These services are more specialised. The PCT is expected to ensure provision of these services somehow, but not all practices will offer everything. These services comprise things such as care of violent patients, minor surgery and flu immunisations.

4. National enhanced services

The PCT itself will decide whether to provide these services. This category covers services such as drug misuse services, anticoagulant services, intrapartum care.

5. Local enhanced services

These services are tailored to local needs, eg care of refugees.

Payment

All practices will receive a 'Global sum' and money for quality payments. This is paid by the Government to the PCT and is ring-fenced so that practices are guaranteed to receive it. The Global sum makes up two-thirds of GPs' payments and comprises payments for essential and additional/enhanced services. Quality payments make up the other third. Quality payments are not paid via the PCT and are separate from the Global sum.

There are six 'quality domains', all offering a potential 1000 points: clinical (eg chronic disease such as asthma, mental health, CHD, diabetes); organisational (education and training, record keeping, practice and medicines management); patient experience (eg length of consultation, patient satisfaction); additional service quality payments (eg achieving a certain percentage uptake of smears); holistic (for achieving across the clinical domain); and quality practice payments (for achieving across the other three domains). Achieving the 48-h access target can make the practice an additional 50 points. Does not apply to quality payments.

Problem with quality payments

Under the QOF, disease prevalence for the ten disease areas in the clinical domain is used to define its workload and is termed the 'prevalence factor'.

Taking this into account when calculating the quality rewards recognises the different amount of work one practice may face in achieving the same number of quality points as another. Originally, it was proposed that quality payments would be made according to the percent of target outcomes achieved, eg HbA1c targets. This, however, fails to take into account disease prevalence. For example, a GP practice in the East End of London whose population has a high prevalence of diabetes would have to work much harder to get their quality payment than a practice serving an affluent population with a low prevalence of diabetes.

For the 2004–5 QOF this failing was addressed by applying a formula. The disease register data are automatically extracted from your clinical systems at the same time as all other contractors by the new Quality and Outcomes Framework Management and Analysis System (QMAS). QMAS aggregates the figures to calculate the national recorded prevalence for each disease area and then adjusts these figures.

First the practice's raw disease prevalence is calculated. This simple formula divides the number of patients on your practice's relevant disease register by the number of patients on the registered list. This gives a 'raw' disease prevalence factor. An adjustment formula is then applied to the raw figure to arrive at the adjusted disease prevalence factor or ADPF.

A cut-off point of 5% is applied to the national range so bringing all contractors at the bottom of the range up to the base level of 5%.

Then, the square root of each practice's prevalence figure is calculated in order to narrow the range of figures. This simply pushes the highest down the range towards the middle and pushes the lowest slightly up. Using the square root is a way of narrowing the national range of disease prevalence. This is because square roots for low numbers are relatively high, and square roots for high numbers are relatively low.

Starting the range at 5% for those practices who have come under this level, and then compressing the range recognises that even practices with relatively low disease prevalence still have costs in setting up registers, buying equipment and monitoring patients.

Using 'raw' prevalence data to calculate financial reward would seriously affect the finances of practices with relatively low prevalence. This goes some way to re-address the balance that the QOF failed to solve in the first year of application.

Management in general practice: the challenge of the new General Medical Services (*Br J Gen Prac* 2004; **54 507**: 734–739)

Managers in general practice perform a variety of roles, from purely administrative to higher-level strategic planning. The aim of this study was to improve understanding of the roles performed by managers in general practice and to consider the implications of this for the implementation of the new GMS contract.

- ✓ In-depth qualitative case studies covering the period before and immediately after the vote in favour of the new GMS contract.

- ✓ Semi-structured interviews with all clinical and managerial personnel in each practice, participant and non-participant observation, and examination of documents.

- ✓ Those practices in the study that employed a manager to work at a strategic level with input into the direction of the organisation demonstrated significant problems with this in practice. These included lack of clarity about what the legitimate role of the manager involved, problems relating to the authority of managers in the context of a partnership, and lack of time available to them to do higher-level work. In addition, general practitioners (GPs) were not confident about their ability to manage their managers' performance.

- ✓ They concluded the new GMS contract will place significant demands on practice management.

These results suggest that it cannot be assumed that simply employing a manager with high-level skills will enable these demands to be met.

Rationing

Know examples of scenarios where rationing may affect your practice, moral obligations, duty of care, postcode prescribing, etc. For example, sildenafil (Viagra®) and donepezil (Aricept®). What in your practice do you not prescribe to certain patients because of cost rather than doubt over clinical efficacy?

Rationing is regarded by many as the only method open if the NHS is to survive while delivering an apparently high standard of publicly funded quality care to the masses.

✓ With rationing you could either deliver the 'best to most' or the 'average to all'; what choice would you make?

✓ The general consensus is that the 'best to most' strategy is the best solution, while still maintaining honesty and transparency to the public.

In New Zealand, a government-appointed committee made a broad assessment of treatment priorities, as in the USA involving the public. It initiated a programme to devise guidelines for the provision of services. Criteria were written to determine access to publicly funded elective surgery. Treatment is given on the ability of patients to benefit (clinically and socially): those with highest need would go first and those with little need may be refused. The obvious disadvantage of either system is that the wealthy could bypass it altogether and hence a two-tier system would be (and has been) created. The poor do not have that option.

Would a modest charge, say, to see a GP help? The answer is 'Yes'. Evidence shows this leads to a reduction in help-seeking behaviour to raise income tax and/or National Insurance (NI) contributions. Hopefully, evidence-based practice and guidelines from NICE will help avoid implicit rationing.

1. Ethical principles and the rationing of health care: a qualitative study in general practice (*Br J Gen Prac* 2005; **55**: 620–625)

Researching sensitive topics, such as the rationing of treatments and denial of care, raises a number of ethical and methodological problems. The study aimed to describe the way in which the allocation of scarce resources is perceived and addressed implicitly and explicitly by GPs in consultations with patients.

✓ A small-scale qualitative study involving purposive sampling, semi-structured interviews and focus groups.

✓ Twenty-four GPs from two contrasting areas of London: one relatively affluent and one relatively deprived.

✓ Initial interviews asked GPs to identify key resource allocation issues.

✓ Analysis of the focus group discussions used 'Doyal's Model'.

While a number of other theoretical models for resource allocation exist, Doyal's model specifically concerns principles of just resource allocation within the NHS. It is related to the moral belief that resources should be allocated on the basis of equal need.

Doyal argues that the substantive principles for ethical decision making within the NHS are:

- ✓ Health care needs should be met in proportion to their distribution within the population.

- ✓ Within areas of treatment, resources should be prioritised on the basis of extremity of need.

- ✓ Those in morally similar need should have an equal chance of access to health care.

- ✓ Scarce resources should not be provided for ineffective health care.

- ✓ Lifestyle should not determine access to health care.

The procedural part to Doyal's framework states that:

- ✓ The public should advise but not determine policy concerning the allocation of health care.

- ✓ Healthcare rationing should be explicit.

In focus group discussions, GPs were given a number of these vignettes to debate.

In conclusion:

- ✓ The use of Doyal's model informed this study in two ways:

1. The principles were used as a standard to measure the ways in which practice conformed or deviated from the ethical principles.

2. GPs are clearly aware of the need for an ethical basis to healthcare rationing, but the realities of the external constraints that they have to work under means that this ethical basis is moderated by the daily necessities inherent in running a surgery.

- ✓ Discussion within the focus groups confirmed wide agreement on general principles of equitable resource allocation, consistent with Doyal's model.

- ✓ Existence of such agreement on principles did little to solve the problem of how more difficult and troubling cases should be resolved.

- ✓ It was recognised that it was often the case that social and psychological factors had a bearing on their decisions.

✓ Factors such as the character of the patient, the consultation style of the doctor, the doctor–patient relationship and the organisational set-up of the practice are all held to have an influence.

While at some general level GPs did accept basic moral principles of fairness and equality as regards the distribution of scarce NHS resources, in practice they were sometimes not aware of the ethical principles they used in decision making or what criteria they employed when priority-setting.

Access to healthcare

The next few sections deal with various innovations in general practice that have to some degree changed the way we see patients and ultimately have improved access.

Access to healthcare over the next few years is likely to dominate the political and primary care arenas. The endpoint is unclear but some expansion of extended GP surgery opening and greater access provision are more than likely to dominate. Having given up our 24-h responsibility it is evident we are going back to a greater or lesser degree to what we have had before. The next paper deals with the impact of some of these changes and their effectiveness on healthcare delivery.

Systematic review of recent innovations in service provision to improve access to primary care (*Br J Gen Prac* 2004; **54**: 374–381)

✓ Access is difficult to define and there is no consensus as to what constitutes 'appropriate' access and what indicates a high degree of access. In general terms, good access exists when patients can get 'the right service at the right time in the right place'. By this definition, utilisation demonstrates people's command over appropriate healthcare resources, which allows them to preserve or improve their health.

✓ Systematic search methods were used to locate random controlled trials (RCTs), systematic reviews, analytical intervention and observational studies conducted in the UK over the last 20 years that provided evidence of seven recent innovations in service provision to improve access or equity, those being:

1. Personal medical services (PMS)

2. GP telephone consultations in general practice

3. Nurse-led telephone consultations in general practice

4. Nurse-led care

5. Walk-in centres

6. NHS Direct

7. Pharmacist led initiatives.

✓ Some evidence to suggest that access is improved by changing the ways in which primary care is delivered.

✓ First-wave PMS pilots facilitated improvements in access to primary care in previously under-served areas.

✓ Walk-in centres and NHS Direct have provided additional access to primary care for white middle-class patients; there is some evidence suggesting that these innovations have increased access inequalities.

✓ There is some evidence that telephone consultations with GPs or nurses can safely substitute face-to-face consultations, although it is not clear that this reduces the number of face-to-face consultations over time.

✓ Nurse practitioners and community pharmacists can manage common conditions without the patient consulting a GP.

✓ Very little robust evidence was found on these innovations; it was insufficiently powerful to determine what does or does not work but provided illumination of a number of innovations that some of us now take for granted.

They concluded that the evidence is insufficient to make clear recommendations regarding ways to improve access to primary care.

NHS Direct

Nurse-led, 24-h telephone helpline has been available throughout England and Wales since the end of 2000.

In response to

- ✓ Growth of the 24-h society
- ✓ Increasing demand for primary and emergency care
- ✓ Problems in recruiting and retaining nurses and general practitioners.

Aims to

- ✓ Reduce workload
- ✓ Provide easy access to an appropriate level of expertise
- ✓ Empower patients with knowledge and thus foster self-care.

Long-term aims

- ✓ Health promotion
- ✓ Information centres
- ✓ Health guides
- ✓ Internet services.

Concerns

- ✓ It will uncover unmet demand, so fuelling workload.
- ✓ Will threaten continuity of care.
- ✓ Telephone contact by nurses rather than a consultation with a GP may mean that important diagnoses are missed.
- ✓ It will not be integrated with the rest of gateway services such as GP cooperatives.
- ✓ Would result in waste of resources and patient confusion.

Criticisms

✓ Service needs to be equally accessible to those without English as a first language, mentally ill people and elderly – they are less likely to use a telephone service.

✓ Money for NHS Direct was not offered to existing primary care services to update the existing service arrangements.

✓ Lack of consistent advice in clinically identical cases.

1. The impact of NHS Direct on the demand for out-of-hours primary and emergency care (*Br J Gen Prac* 2005; **55**: 790–792)

There is considerable evidence that demand for out-of-hours primary care in the UK has been rising for many years. In the past 15 years this has resulted in a number of major changes to the provision of out-of-hours care, including the development of GP cooperatives and, in 1998, the creation of NHS Direct.

✓ Study undertook a national study to determine whether NHS Direct helped to control rising demand for out-of-hours primary and emergency care during its first 3 years of operation.

✓ During its first 3 years, NHS Direct handled 5,180,000 calls in England.

✓ This analysis of the impact of successive waves of NHS Direct in England and Wales suggests that it has reduced calls to out-of-hours general practice, reversing the previous upward trend, but has had a negligible impact on the volume of demand for emergency ambulance services and hospital emergency departments.

✓ For the 'average cooperative', the mean effect was equivalent to a reduction of about seven calls per night, over the first year, becoming greater in subsequent years.

✓ Non-response and missing data limit the study, but the authors state that response bias is unlikely to have had any important impact on our results.

✓ The number of patients seen in person may have remained constant, or even increased, but to resolve this question would require more detailed studies.

2. NHS Direct versus general practice based triage for same day appointments in primary care: cluster randomised controlled trial (*BMJ* 2004; **329**: 774)

The objective of this study was to assess the relative effects on consultation workload and costs of off-site triage by NHS Direct for patients requesting same-day appointments compared with usual on-site nurse telephone triage in general practice.

- ✓ Cluster RCT involving three primary care sites in York, England.

- ✓ 4703 patients: 2452 with practice-based triage, 2251 with NHS Direct triage.

- ✓ Outcome measures were the type of consultation after request for same-day appointment (telephone, appointment, or visit); time taken for consultation; service use during the month after same-day contact; costs of same-day, follow-up and emergency care.

- ✓ The results showed patients in the NHS Direct group were less likely to have their call resolved by a nurse and were more likely to have an appointment with a general practitioner.

- ✓ Mean total time per patient in the NHS Direct group was 7.62 min longer than in the practice-based group.

- ✓ Costs were greater in the NHS Direct group — £2.88 (£0.88 to £4.87) per patient triaged — as a result of the difference between the groups in proportions of patients at each final point of contact after triage.

The authors concluded that external management of requests for same-day appointments by nurse telephone triage through NHS Direct is possible but comes at a higher cost than practice-nurse-delivered triage in primary care. If NHS Direct could achieve the same proportions of consultation types as practice-based triage, costs would be comparable.

3. National Audit Office Report published January 2002

- ✓ Stated – NHS Direct is used less by ethnic minorities, people aged over 65 years and disadvantaged groups than by the general population.

- ✓ Report stated that these groups had 'as much need as others and perhaps an even greater one'.

✓ Service has also reduced demand on healthcare services that are provided outside normal working hours, eg GPs.

✓ One GP cooperative providing out-of-hours services saw an 18% fall in the number of calls received when callers were transferred to NHS Direct first.

Walk-in Centres

✓ Announced in April 1999

✓ Offer people the opportunity to see a healthcare professional face to face on a walk-in basis.

✓ Open weekdays and weekends to provide information and treatment for minor conditions.

✓ Sited in convenient locations, mainly in large towns.

✓ Consultations mainly provided by nurses, using clinical assessment software.

✓ These nurse-led centres provide advice and treatment for minor illnesses and also direct people to the most appropriate healthcare provider for their needs.

✓ Same concerns voiced over NHS Direct have been discussed with regard to Walk-in centres.

✓ Run by cooperatives, GPs and NHS Trusts.

Objections

✓ Diversion of funds from other parts of primary care.

✓ May generate additional demands.

✓ May cause fragmentation of primary care and erosion of Family Doctor Service which has:

- Comprehensive medical record

- Continuity of care at its core

- Gatekeeper role.

Benefits

✓ May reduce workload of GPs (especially trivial).

✓ Responds to demand for wider access.

✓ NHS Direct may help the public make more appropriate use of health and social services.

 1. An observational study comparing quality of care in Walk-in centres with general practice and NHS Direct using standardised patients (*BMJ* 2002; **324**: 1556)

In this observational study there was direct comparison of quality of clinical care in Walk-in centres with that provided in general practice and by NHS Direct.

✓ Outcome measures were mean scores on consensus-derived checklists of essential items for the management of the clinical scenarios.

✓ Data were also collected on access to and referral by Walk-in centres, general practices and NHS Direct.

✓ Walk-in centres achieved a significantly greater mean score for all scenarios combined than general practices and NHS Direct.

✓ Walk-in centres performed particularly well on postcoital contraception and asthma scenarios. In contrast to general practice, Walk-in centres and NHS Direct referred a higher proportion of patients.

✓ They performed significantly less well than general practice in examination of chest pain and the diagnosis, advice and treatment of sinusitis.

✓ Walk-in centres' better performance was particularly noticeable for history taking, perhaps owing to the longer consultations undertaken in this setting.

The authors concluded that Walk-in centres perform adequately and safely compared with general practices and NHS Direct for the range of conditions under study, but the impact of referrals on workload of other healthcare providers requires further research.

Problems

✓ Non-random sampling of participating sites.

✓ Use of a limited number of scenarios, some of which are more discriminating than others.

✓ Participating sites, particularly general practices, were likely to be more interested in the research question and may have provided a higher quality of care.

✓ Scenarios were chosen as typical of those seen in Walk-in centres and because they were appropriate for portrayal by standardised patients.

✓ Scenarios necessitating the presence of abnormal findings or potentially involving certain types of physical examination or referral to third parties could not be included.

2. Questionnaire survey of users of NHS Walk-in centres: observational study (Br J Gen Pract 2002; 52: 554–561)

This study attempted, through a questionnaire, to ascertain the client group that attended and their satisfaction.

✓ The survey was also conducted among people who attended general practices close to a Walk-in centre on a 'same-day' basis.

✓ For this group of people, attending a nearby Walk-in centre would be a realistic alternative source of care.

✓ The questionnaire was divided into two sections. The first was designed to be completed before the consultation and included questions about sociodemographic characteristics, convenience of location and opening hours, reasons for consulting, expectations, recent use of health services and attitudes to continuity of care. The second section, completed after the consultation, included questions about waiting times, satisfaction, treatment, referrals and enablement.

✓ The results showed that, compared to GP visitors, Walk-in centre visitors were more likely to:

- Be owner-occupiers (55% vs 49%)

- Have further education (25% vs 19%)

- Be Caucasian (88% vs 84%).

✓ Main reasons for attending a Walk-in centre were speed of access and convenience.

✓ Walk-in centre visitors were more likely to attend on the first day of illness (28% vs 10%).

✓ Walk-in centre visitors were less likely to expect a prescription (38% vs 70%) and placed less importance on continuity.

✓ People were more satisfied with Walk-in centres than with general practice.

They concluded that NHS Walk-in centres improve access to care, but not necessarily for those people with the greatest health needs as visitors to Walk-in centres were younger, better educated and more affluent than those attending general practice.

Diagnostic and treatment centres

The Government is planning to commission certain services to private clinics, which will be staffed by local or foreign doctors. One hundred and forty thousand operations such as cataract extraction and hip and knee surgery are planned each year. The stated aim is to take the pressure off NHS facilities, reduce waiting times and allow hospitals to 'focus their expertise' on complicated elective work. However, there has been concern regarding the following points.

These centres may not be cost-effective

Many hospitals have already spent money to try to cut waiting times by increasing staff and facilities. If patients are diverted away to private clinics, there may have to be job losses. Often, routine operations such as cataract extraction help hospitals to subsidise more specialised work, eg in chronic eye disease. Posts which do not offer enough experience for surgical trainees will be taken away, potentially leaving consultants without junior staff. Surgical trainees may get insufficient experience of routine surgery. Also follow-up arrangements for patients may not be comparable.

Public–private partnerships appear to be generally popular with this Government. For example, hospitals are being built under 'PFIs' (private finance initiatives). The LIFT scheme (Local Improvement Finance Trust) is a PFI and is going to put £1 billion into building new premises in deprived areas; PCTs bid for pots of money, which go into local schemes. There are obviously concerns about the motivation of the private companies involved and about long-term consequences and costs to the NHS.

Specialist GPs

In January 2004, there were 1250 specialist GPs practising in the UK (the *NHS Plan* stated that there should be 1000 in place by 2004). Key points regarding the benefits and threats of the new grade were raised.

Potential benefits

✓ Getting high-quality care more rapidly and closer to home offers patients considerable advantages.

✓ Increased communication between local GPs may enhance team working and continuity.

✓ Clinical care outside general practice also offers interest, personal development and heightened self-esteem for GPs.

✓ Advantages for GPs may include enhanced retention, delayed burnout and increased job satisfaction.

✓ Increased working with consultants will also help to break down barriers.

Potential threats

✓ The creation of GPs with special interests may degrade the discipline of general practice and the value of generalism.

✓ Fragmentation of general practice, with the devaluing and eventual loss of generalism, to the detriment of patient care, as has occurred with general physicians.

✓ Adverse effects on resources.

✓ Specialist GPs may become a second-class service designed to ease the pressure on hospital outpatient clinics, reducing clinical standards while denying patient access.

USEFUL WEBSITE

'General Practitioners With Special Interests' is accessible at www.rcgp.org.uk

Nurse practitioners

What work might they do?

✓ Prevention, immunisation, smears, contraception, review BP, asthma, diabetes, etc.

✓ Medical triage, independent management of minor illness with limited prescribing rights, referring to GP only when necessary.

✓ Social triage – guiding patients needing social or financial help.

How would GPs benefit?

✓ Overtrained for much of what we do – less time spent on trivia would mean that more time is available for patients with more serious problems.

✓ Skills learnt during training need no longer atrophy through disuse.

✓ Potential for GPs to specialise in aspects of primary care.

✓ Increased job satisfaction.

✓ Increased income through larger lists, eg 4000 patients per doctor.

What are the possible problems?

✓ Dilution of continuity of care and of personal care.

✓ GPs may feel themselves redundant.

✓ Nurses may fail to diagnose rare but life-threatening conditions, or to spot unusual presentations.

✓ More specialisation by GPs may lead to loss of 'generalist role'.

✓ Legal responsibility – nurses are responsible for own actions but GPs still have 'vicarious liability'.

What do the studies show?

Nurse practitioners are

- ✓ Safe
- ✓ Effective
- ✓ Popular with patients
- ✓ Good at listening, understanding and explaining
- ✓ Good at following protocols
- ✓ Less likely to prescribe
- ✓ More likely to use non-prescription approaches
- ✓ Likely to advise on prevention
- ✓ Good at using drug formularies.

What are the pitfalls?

(This is food for thought, not necessarily the authors' views)

- ✓ The title 'Nurse Practitioner' is not regulated, the courses they go on are neither externally assessed nor regulated.
- ✓ Are we therefore allowing non-medically trained people to practise as doctors?
- ✓ Having to access a GP only via a nurse, is it acceptable that patients do not have a choice to see a doctor first.
- ✓ Introduction of a two-tier service with nurses providing much of the care in those areas where it is difficult to recruit GPs.
- ✓ What effect would it have on the nature of general practice?
- ✓ Ability to distinguish self-limiting from serious disease and the opportunity to develop a close rapport with patients are key skills of GPs, would these be compromised?

1. Survey of the impact of nurse telephone triage on general practitioner (Br J Gen Prac, 2004; **54 500**: 207–210)

The effect of nurse telephone triage on workload has been reported in a number of trials. This study investigated doctors' perceptions by surveying the impact of this new same-day appointment management system on GPs' consulting behaviours.

- ✓ Survey of GP consultations was carried out in three surgery sites operated by a large general practice in inner city York.

- ✓ Six practice nurses, who had received 30 hours of minor illness management training and were supported by a number of computerised management protocols developed by the practice, conducted a telephone assessment of all patients requesting same-day appointments.

- ✓ Following triage, patients received one of the following: telephone advice only from the nurse or GP, a same-day nurse appointment, a same-day GP appointment, a home visit, or a routine nurse or GP appointment.

- ✓ In the triage system, patients had more presenting problems and GP consultation behaviours were greater on three out of the four other indicators, requiring more consultations, prescription items and investigations per patient.

- ✓ The rate of referral to secondary care was unchanged.

- ✓ This survey concludes that GPs working in practices with nurse telephone triage systems behave as if their caseloads are more challenging.

- ✓ GPs identified more presenting problems per patient and increased their consulting behaviours on three out of four activity indicators: consultations, prescriptions and investigations.

- ✓ Differences between the two groups of patients on the indicators may be regarded as quite small, but they were clearly noticeable and clinically significant.

✓ The study implies that changes to the mixture of skills in primary care, where nurses are used in managing some same-day appointments, may result in the need for GPs to change their consulting behaviours to accommodate an increase in the mean number of problems presented per patient, as those patients with self-limiting illnesses are seen elsewhere in the primary care team. Nurse telephone triage reduces the number of extra same-day appointment requests that have to be fitted into GPs' surgeries by 40%.

2. Nurse management of patients with minor illnesses in general practice: a multicentre RCT (*BMJ* 2000; **320**: 1038)

This article explored the changing roles of nurses in the NHS. Four trials of nurse impact on primary care were published. Practice nurses attended a degree-level course on managing minor illness for half a day a week for three months, they also observed GPs in surgeries twice a week. Two sessions equates to one day or two surgery lists. Two-month pilot period after the nurses were recruited.

✓ Patients asking for same-day appointments with minor illness were randomly distributed between a GP and practice nurse.

✓ High satisfaction for both doctor and nurse consultations (but significantly higher for nurses).

✓ Consultations with nurses took an average of 10 min, with doctors 8 min.

✓ Similar prescription rates for a similar number of patients.

✓ 73% of patients seen by nurses required no input from doctors.

✓ Conclusion – practice nurses offer an effective service for people with minor illness.

3. Impact of nurse practitioners on workload of general practitioners: randomised controlled trial (*BMJ* 2004; **328**: 927)

This study from the Netherlands examined the impact on GP's workload of adding nurse practitioners to the general practice team.

- ✓ RCT with measurements before and after the introduction of nurse practitioners.

- ✓ Five nurses were randomly allocated to GPs to undertake specific elements of care according to agreed guidelines. The control group received no nurse.

- ✓ Outcome was measured by objective workload, derived from 28-day diaries, included the number of contacts per day for each of three conditions (chronic obstructive pulmonary disease or asthma, dementia, cancer), by type of consultation and by time of day.

- ✓ Subjective workload was measured by using a validated questionnaire.

- ✓ Results showed the number of contacts during surgery hours increased in the intervention group compared with the control group, particularly for patients with chronic obstructive pulmonary disease or asthma.

- ✓ The number of consultations out of hours declined slightly in the intervention group compared with the control group.

- ✓ No significant changes became apparent in subjective workload.

The authors concluded that adding nurse practitioners to general practice teams did not reduce the workload of GPs; at least in the short term. Nurse practitioners are used as supplements, rather than substitutes, for care given by general practitioners.

Post 'Shipman': what are the long-term effects?

There has been a wide-ranging inquiry into the issues raised by the case. Following the publication of the inquiry into the Shipman case it appears that Harold Shipman murdered at least 215 of his patients (171 women and 44 men): 45 other cases are possibly suspicious. The head of the inquiry, High

Court Judge Dame Janet Smith, also speculated that Shipman may have been hoping to get caught when he altered the will of his last victim, Kathleen Grundy, aged 81 years. The forgery was described as 'crude' and 'made detection inevitable'.

Harold Shipman committed suicide in January 2004 and admitted guilt in a letter to his wife before he died. Dame Janet Smith recommended changes to the current systems, in a report published in July 2003.

- ✓ She heavily criticised the current system of death certification, in that it relies too much on the integrity of a single doctor.

- ✓ She has proposed that all deaths be referred to a coroner's service – a combination of medical coroners, judicial coroners and coroner's investigators.

- ✓ Where a doctor has been able to give an opinion on the cause of death, a coroner's investigator will look into the case and certify death. If not, the medical coroners will look into the case in more detail.

- ✓ In all cases, the investigator will talk to the family of the deceased to find possible inconsistencies in the GP's story.

- ✓ GPs will have to complete a new form 2, giving an account of the circumstances leading up to death, a brief medical history and details of nursing care. They will no longer certify death and there will be no separate cremation form.

- ✓ Dame Janet wants the GMC to impose an ethical professional duty on doctors to cooperate. The BMA has welcomed Dame Smith's proposals, but there is serious concern about time and staffing issues.

USEFUL WEBSITE

www.the-shipman-inquiry.org.uk/reports.asp – Shipman Inquiry reports

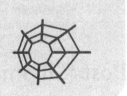

Possible effects of the case on single-handed/small practices

- ✓ Profession should be defending single-handed practices

- ✓ Professional isolation should be the focus

- ✓ Restore patient confidence by professional development, revalidation and appraisal

- ✓ Death rates, although crude, may become part of any clinical governance monitoring system

- ✓ Stricter control of use and storage of controlled drugs.

1. Editorial: The future of single-handed general practices
(*BMJ* 2005; **330**: 1460–1461)

This editorial focused on the apparent decline of single-handed practices and the possible reasons for the change. Ever since the foundation of the NHS, single-handed general practitioners have made an important contribution in the UK, particularly in inner city and rural areas where recruiting general practitioners has proved difficult.

- ✓ Between 1994 and 2003, the number of single-handed general practitioners fell from 2959 to 2578 (from 10.8% to 8.5% of all general practitioners) in England.

- ✓ Between 2003 and 2004, the number fell by a further 660 to 1918 (now comprising 6.1%).

- ✓ Doctors may also find larger practices more attractive to work in because they reduce the likelihood of clinical isolation, can employ more support staff, allow scope for specialisation, and offer a wider range of services than small practices.

- ✓ However, a more important reason for the decline in the number of small practices could be that they might not feature in the UK government's long-term vision for primary care.

- ✓ Small practices are seen as less efficient and more difficult to manage by many policy makers and managers.

- ✓ The Shipman case may also have contributed to this desire to reshape general practice.

✓ Among the recommendations arising from the Shipman inquiry was that the NHS should take steps to reduce the clinical isolation of single-handed practitioners.

Studies that have compared the quality of care in smaller practices with that in larger practices have found little relation between practice size and quality. Smaller practices are considered by patients to be more accessible and achieve higher levels of satisfaction among patients than larger practices.

Practice-based commissioning

GP practices holding budgets for the care of their patients is far from a new ideal. Fund-holding in its day offered similar scope and innovation. The key differences may well be based on who profits from the process, whether that is the GPs, patients or both, and the public perception it will carry.

In 1998 the white paper The New NHS stated 'the Government expects PCTs will extend indicative budgets to individual practices for the full range of services'.

In June of 2004, The NHS Improvement Plan indicated that, 'from April 2005, GP practices that wish to do so will be given indicative commissioning budgets'.

Fund-holding was seen by many as providing extra profit for doctors whereas practice-based commissioning (PBC) with its restrictions on where and how savings are spent does not.

PBC is seen as entirely consistent with the principle of greater devolution.

The effects on the NHS and GP practices of the introduction of PBC are as yet not clear. However, there are some changes which are almost certain:

✓ PBC will be a driver for quality, empowerment and service innovation.

✓ Practices will be able to commission a wider range of services, from more providers, that are close to homes of patients and essentially more convenient.

✓ Patients will be able to choose when and where to have their treatment and procedures (ie The Choice Agenda and Choose & Book).

✓ From 2008, patients will have free choice for elective procedures.

✓ Practices could then use their commissioning abilities to identify provision (including primary care and private or independent sector providers) to give patients more choice.

✓ It will be in the practices' interests to develop an extended range of services that may defer input to Acute Trusts and offer the patient more choice.

✓ Payment by results (PBR) will mean the payment for the procedure undertaken will follow the patient. In reality it is envisaged a patient will have a choice of multiple providers including GP-led services, the independent sector and the Acute Trusts and the payment will go to whomever the patient chooses. This is therefore an internal competitive market within the NHS.

✓ There is also emphasis placed on managing long-term illness with more substantive care packages that would be efficiently provided through careful management and competition between providers.

The indicative budget

Every practice will ultimately receive statements annually regarding its performance on the use of services and the costs of them. It already occurs for prescribing and some others services depending on location. However all PCTs will have to provide this service covering all aspects of care, including prescribing, scheduled care, unscheduled care and diagnostics. PCTs will be judged by the DoH on their relative abilities to provide this service.

The indicative budget is not a cheque of money to the practice but represents your share of the PCTs budget that you will manage.

From this money, with the PCT's support, practices or groups of practices will identify health needs for which to commission and develop new services. The GPs as commissioners will then get the PCT (as contractors) to develop the service.

The PCT would continue to hold the actual budget and will remain responsible for the contracts with the secondary care provider.

Savings from efficiency may only be used for patient services with the exception of management costs that are needed to drive the process.

Over the next three years practices will move towards holding budgets covering the entire scope of health care provision, except for some highly specialised or cross-PCT services such as Mental Health in some localities.

Practice groups

In order for practices to manage their budget it has also been necessary for smaller practices to group together to have larger collective list sizes and therefore budgets so that variances can be minimised. It will then also allow them perhaps to employ staff across the practices which makes more financial sense. It is not unforeseeable that practices may even employ consultants to their groups for the provision of services.

The risks

The budget until 2008 will be risk managed by the PCT; in essence, this means if the practice overspends then the risk lies with the PCT rather than the GPs. The practices will be expected to at least balance their budgets over the next three years. If they are unable to do so then they will risk forfeiting the right to hold an indicative budget except in exceptional circumstances. These may include high isolated expensive cases, mergers of poorly performing practices with plans in place to demonstrate improvement or evidence they have previously balanced the budget. However the situation when it arises remains far from clear.

The bigger risk is that practices will be put off by the process or not see sufficient reward for undertaking what is a large and complex task. The risk of not participating is that organisations have already started to form to take practice's budgets and manage them. This may lead to the situation that GP practices will be managed by an external entity wholly and completely. Ultimately, this may mean over the longer term more GPs becoming salaried as opposed to principles.

From 2008 Foundation Trusts as well as other private sector companies will be able to enter the primary care arena. The competitive process that PBC will bring to secondary care will then enter primary care. The effect of this is uncertain and unknown. What can be said is that GPs' assumption that they remain the sole gatekeepers is certainly and definitely under threat of change.

The National Programme for Information Technology (NPfIT)

With so much change and so many acronyms being created daily it is sometimes hard to keep up with what may really be innovative and what appears to be over bureaucratic nonsense. NPfIT promises much and the potential for real change is vast. I by no means extend the virtues for or against this scheme but would advise you read, become aware and form your own opinion on what may be fundamental to the existence of General Practice as the majority of us know it, but not what the DoH has planned for us.

The National Programme for Information Technology (NPfIT)
(*Br J Gen Prac* 2005; **55**: 85–86)

The GP as gatekeeper – a bastion worth fighting for? This editorial considers the need and rationale behind the NHS's IT policy. In Summary:

- ✓ The National Programme for Information Technology (NPfIT) has the potential to change forever the way in which health care is provided.

- ✓ Governments are beginning to realise that the utilisation of modern technologies is necessary in order to cope with these growing demands.

- ✓ GPs' majors concerns revolve around the impact of NPfIT on choice of systems and potential disruption to current service.

- ✓ However, it needs to be stressed that NPfIT is about more than software but the vision of a health service that is different to that which we know today.

- ✓ NPfIT is driven by a political agenda to change health care.

- ✓ One of the main objectives for primary care is the 'supermarket' approach. A patient can select which service they want to use from a variety of general practices, Walk-in centres, and privately provided and specialist services, and information systems are seen as the catalyst to this, as anyone can provide care given that they have access to the records.

- ✓ A logical conclusion from this is that the GP will no longer act as 'gatekeeper'.

✓ This new-found freedom provides patients with a staggering range of choice.

✓ The advent of NPfIT has the potential to create a single, comprehensive patient record, accessible by both patient and physician.

✓ NPfIT is likely to improve the availability of patient records, but will this improve patient care?

✓ The experience in countries where primary care is provided by direct access to specialists shows that patients often do not go to the right specialist.

✓ Choice may sound like a good thing, but when you are ill you need a friend who will make decisions both for and with you.

✓ While the NPfIT is lauded by many, the author remains unconvinced that its impact on patients and professionals has really been considered and addressed.

Therefore, perhaps it is best for GPs to stand fast in their role as patient advocates, and to work together with patients and other professionals to ensure that the good within the health service is not undone while excising the bad.

CHAPTER 13: MEDICINE AND THE INTERNET

CHAPTER 13:
MEDICINE AND THE INTERNET

The internet is a fast growing source of health information and support for patients. Typing the word 'health' into a well-known search engine will throw up over 286 million relevant websites!

Increasingly, patients are now using the internet to search for detailed information about their medical condition; they can obtain a second opinion from a 'cyberdoc' and can also check with various patient support groups about their best treatment options. The knowledge gained can then be used to challenge their doctor during subsequent consultations, which may then affect the doctor–patient relationship. Recent surveys have shown that 40–54% of patients access medical information via the internet and that this information affects their choice of treatment.

What makes the internet attractive?

As part of their everyday work, doctors and other healthcare professionals need to access information. The internet accelerates and broadens such provision. Patients, too, often want more information and they can search for remedies on the internet. Medical information is thought to be one of the most retrieved types of information on the internet. Through the internet, patients not only have access to almost as much information as clinicians, but they are also starting to provide advice to other patients through websites that they host and manage. Even children can provide information to their peers, their parents and clinicians.

A study has shown that accessing information and/or support online can have a profound effect on men's experiences of prostate cancer (*Qual Health Res* 2005; **15**: 325). It can provide a method of taking some control over their disease and limiting inhibitions experienced in face-to-face encounters.

People with cancer have been shown to use the internet for a wide range of information and support needs at many different stages of their illness (*BMJ* 2004; **328**: 577).

Is there any regulation of the information available on the internet?

A major concern is the reliability of the information accessed, opinions offered, claims made and materials supplied by the internet. The quality of websites varies tremendously. One study found that providing references to scientific publications or prescribing information was significantly associated with high content quality (*Br J Clin Pharmacol* 2004; **57**: 80).

What is the Health on the Net Foundation?

Health on the Net Foundation (see website) is an international, non-profit-making organisation based in Geneva. It provides a database of evaluated health materials, and also promotes the use of the HON code as a self-governance initiative to help unify the quality of medical and health information available. Users of website health information displaying the HON logo can be assured that the material has been developed in accordance with these guidelines. This is the oldest, and probably best known, quality label.

What problems may the internet pose to healthcare professionals?

Although data are not yet available, it is evident that clinicians can find themselves upstaged by and ill-prepared to cope with those patients who bring along information downloaded from the internet. More resources are needed to study the implications of the internet for the role of patients and clinicians, and also to ensure that the clinician–patient relationship is strengthened rather than undermined. It has been proposed that public health practitioners and healthcare professionals should be involved in the design, dissemination and evaluation of web-based health and medical information (*Health Promot Int* 2003; **18**: 381).

Problems with the internet include an uneven quality of medical information available, difficulties in finding, understanding and using the information and the potential for harm and risks of over-consumption.

Are there any problems with writing for medical websites?

Doctors are less likely to face criticism for placing medical information on a website, providing it does not refer to specific cases. It is recommended that a statement be added stating that the medical advice provided is as accurate as possible, but should not be used as a substitute for advice that patients can obtain from their own doctors. Technology is increasingly becoming integrated into modern clinical practice, so it is therefore important that all users are fully aware of any of its potential pitfalls.

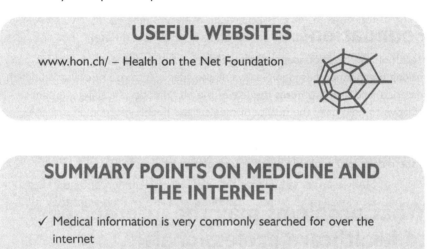

USEFUL WEBSITES

www.hon.ch/ – Health on the Net Foundation

SUMMARY POINTS ON MEDICINE AND THE INTERNET

✓ Medical information is very commonly searched for over the internet

✓ Downloaded information is often very challenging to doctors

✓ Information is often inaccurate

✓ Healthcare professionals should be involved in creating medical websites

The e-patient and e-mail consultations

There appears to be a growing amount of literature in the academic press about a process that has inherently existed by its own means for some time. It clearly appears that the internet-savvy patient is here to stay and that modern medical consultation may involve varying degrees of IT skills as time goes on. Below are a few articles highlighting this growing field.

1. Editorial: The first generation of e-patients *(BMJ* 2004; **328**: 1148–1149)

This interesting article charts the emergence of e-patients and the ramifications it holds for the medical profession. In summary:

- ✓ About half of adults in the USA have looked for health information on the net, making this the third most popular online activity.

- ✓ E-patients (including those who seek online guidance for their own ailments and the friends and family members who go online on their behalf) report two effects of their online health research – 'better health information and services, and different (but not always better) relationships with their doctors'.

- ✓ Firstly, many clinicians have underestimated the benefits and overestimated the risks of online health resources for patients.

- ✓ Reports of patients coming to harm as the result of online advice are rare, whereas accounts of those who have obtained better care, averted medical mistakes, or saved their own lives are common.

- ✓ Many e-patients say that the medical information and guidance they can find online is more complete and useful than what they receive from their clinicians.

- ✓ Medical online support groups have become an important healthcare resource.

- ✓ The net friendliness of clinicians and provider organisations, as rated by the e-patients they serve, is becoming an important new aspect of healthcare quality.

- ✓ When clinicians respond negatively to e-patients' requests to discuss materials they have found online and act as if they feel that their authority is being challenged by such requests, it may damage or disrupt the doctor–patient relationship.

- ✓ Much of the fundamental research in this emerging field remains to be done.

- ✓ The medical world view of the twentieth century did not recognise the legitimacy of lay medical competence and autonomy.

- ✓ Something akin to a major system upgrade in our thinking is needed, a new cultural operating system for healthcare in which e-patients can be recognised as a valuable new type of renewable resource managing much of their own care, providing care for others, helping professionals improve the quality of their services, and participating in collaborations between patients and professionals.

✓ Given the recognition and support they deserve these new medical colleagues may help us find sustainable solutions to the seemingly intractable problems that now plague all modern systems.

2. E-mail consultations in health care: 1 Scope and effectiveness (BMJ 2004; **329**: 435–438)

In the first of a two-article series the authors consider the potential for e-mail consultations and summarise the evidence about their use for preventive healthcare, health education and managing non-urgent conditions. E-mail now represents an integral part of daily life for about 60% of the UK population.

The first article explores the scope for e-mail consultations for preventive health care, health education, and managing non-urgent conditions.

In summary

Potential advantages of e-mail in delivering health care

✓ Increased convenience in time and space for patient and doctor.

✓ May reduce the need for face-to-face consultations.

✓ Useful for information that patients would have to remember or write down if it were given orally (such as addresses and telephone numbers of services, test results with interpretations and advice, instructions on taking drugs).

✓ Unlimited length.

✓ Increased access to care (eg for those with physical disabilities or living in a remote area).

✓ Increased opportunities for information sharing.

✓ User-friendly medium for patients to ask for further clarification after a face-to-face consultation.

✓ Allows patients to discuss content of messages with family or friends to improve understanding.

✓ Free style of writing.

✓ Speed of communication.

✓ Doctors can consult with colleagues and other professionals to provide a more considered response.

✓ Ability to offer routine transactions and patient education information to several people simultaneously.

✓ Potential cost savings.

Potential disadvantages of e-mail use in delivering health care

✓ May widen social disparities by allowing preferential access to wealthier people and young middle class adults.

✓ Like other forms of written communication, e-mail does not easily provide the subtle emotive cues gleaned from vocal intonation and physical demeanour that aid interpretation.

✓ Inability to examine the patient.

✓ May increase the risk of diagnostic or communication errors.

✓ Potential slow responses to messages that might require emergency actions.

✓ Threats to patient privacy.

✓ Providers may be overwhelmed by the volume and length of e-mails.

3. E-mail consultations in health care: 2 Acceptability and safe application (BMJ 2004; 329: 439–442)

In the second article the authors consider the potential for e-mail consultations. E-mail may have an important role in augmenting and facilitating communication between patients and healthcare professionals.

✓ National surveys show that patients increasingly want to be able to communicate with healthcare professionals by e-mail.

✓ However, few doctors currently do so: professional concerns centre on the quality of consultations, confidentiality, liability and the challenge of recovering fees.

✓ Early e-mail use in healthcare has grown without an adequate supporting infrastructure to address security issues.

✓ Ensuring privacy, confidentiality and security of information is vital for e-mail consultations.

✓ E-mail consultations mark a radical shift from the traditional oral modes of communication: both patients and doctors need education in how to use them safely and effectively.

Key features of optimal software for e-mail consultations

1. Ease of adoption (combining with existing technologies).

2. Adaptability to an organisation's unique requirements for managing personal health information.

3. Seamless operating with existing infrastructures.

4. Enabling communication over various operating systems and software programs.

5. User friendliness – easy to set up, manage and use by doctors and patients.

6. Effective, invisible security over wired and wireless environments.

7. Easy authentication methods.

8. Integration with existing medical records systems.

9. Possibility of the use of customised templates for e-mail consultations.

10. Automation functions (such as automatic replies).

11. System for preventing generation of messages to an addressee if previous messages remained unanswered for longer than set permissible time.

12. Integrated customisable message content filtering.

13. Virus scanning.

14. Track and audit messaging system.

15. Archiving and logging.

CHAPTER 14:
COMPLEMENTARY
MEDICINE

CHAPTER 14:
COMPLEMENTARY MEDICINE

Many more people are now using complementary and alternative medicine; up to 10% of NHS physiotherapists are currently using acupuncture. It has been estimated that alternative medicine is used by about 30% of the population in the UK, which is actually much less than in Germany and the USA.

Legally, herbal products are classified as food supplements and are widely available from health food shops and chemists. Currently, it is legal for anyone in the UK to practise alternative medicine without any training (except chiropractic and osteopathy). Many complementary practitioners claim that their treatments are more cost-effective and safer than conventional medicine; however, the evidence for this is still very scanty and weak. Most people quite rightly accept that neither safety nor efficacy can be assumed; any alternative treatment must now be supported by hard evidence. Good design of randomised controlled trials (RCTs) would avoid invalid results and misrepresentation of the holistic essence of complementary medicine.

Patients fear the safety of medicines; especially with scares about adverse effects and withdrawal of some medicines from the market. Patients perceive treatments containing herbal agents to be 'natural' and therefore safe.

A widespread lack of interest in interactions between herbal products and prescribed medicines is putting the public at risk. A study found that most pharmaceutical and herbal companies had never conducted research regarding herb–drug interactions (*Arch Intern Med* 2003; **163**: 1371). The efficacy of herbal medicines has been tested in hundreds of clinical trials which are not all of inferior methodological quality. However, the evidence on herbal medicines is incomplete, complex and confusing (*BMJ* 2003; **327**: 881).

Documented characterisation of herbal supplements in published RCTs is still inadequate. The varying quality of herbs used in trials make conclusions hard to interpret. Of 81 RCTs studied recently, only 12 quantified the actual contents of the herbal preparations used (*Am J Med* 2005; **118**: 1087–1093). Investigators may be unaware of the extent to which herbal quality-control issues may detract from the value of otherwise well-designed clinical trials.

In September 2004, the Medicines and Healthcare Products Regulatory Agency (MHRA) issued a press statement warning consumers that the poor quality of some traditional Chinese medicines can pose a health risk to those using them. In it, they urged consumers not to take a product which is not labelled in English and advised that even the presence of English labelling is not a guarantee of a safe, good-quality product.

The European Directive on Traditional Herbal Medicinal Products has set out clear standards for the safety and quality of over-the-counter traditional herbal medicines.

Practitioners of traditional Chinese medicine have agreed to cooperate with the Department of Health to improve the safety of traditional medicines after concerns that they may contain potentially toxic or carcinogenic ingredients. The Committee on the Safety of Medicines (CSM) have found banned substances such as mercury and arsenic in traditional Chinese medicines sold in the UK, despite previous warnings. Some medicines also contained steroids, even though the label did not declare it. Banned products containing the herb *Aristolochia*, which has been associated with two cases of kidney disease in the UK, are also still being offered for sale.

St John's wort

St John's wort (*Hypericum perforatum*) is an increasingly popular choice for the treatment of depression, and there is plenty of evidence which shows that *Hypericum* is as effective as imipramine in the treatment of mild to moderate depression (*BMJ* 2000; **321**: 536–539). A double-blind randomised clinical trial showed that St John's wort is at least as effective as paroxetine in ameliorating the symptoms of moderately or severely depressed patients (*BMJ* 2005; **330**: 503).

However, the use of St John's wort is more limited than initially thought as it is a liver inducer and therefore reduces levels of digoxin, carbamazepine, warfarin and the oral contraceptive pill. It has numerous interactions with other drugs, which patients should be warned of before starting it.

Ginkgo biloba

The published evidence suggests that ginkgo is of questionable use for treating memory loss and tinnitus, but that it has some effect on both dementia and intermittent claudication (*Ann Intern Med* 2002; **136**: 42–53). It is, however, also a potent inhibitor of platelet-activating factor, so increasing the risk of intracerebral haemorrhage in those people taking aspirin and warfarin.

Phytoestogens

Phytoestrogen supplements have been topical recently in view of the adverse publicity regarding hormone-replacement therapy. However, postmenopausal supplementation with soy protein containing isoflavones does not improve cognitive function or affect bone mineral density or plasma lipids (*JAMA* 2004; **292**: 65). Previous studies evaluating an effect of isoflavones on postmenopausal hot flushes have also found minimal benefit.

Saw Palmetto

Recent evidence suggests that the use of saw palmetto leads to improvements in urinary function for those suffering from benign prostatic hyperplasia (BPH). The favourable comparison of saw palmetto with tamsulosin, a well-known first-line agent in the treatment of urinary tract symptoms, demonstrates promise towards a beneficial effect of this herbal agent, with very few, if any, adverse effects. However, what degree of this beneficial activity is due to placebo effects has yet to be determined. In addition, the precise mechanism of action of saw palmetto in men with BPH remains unclear.

Is there any good evidence available to support homoeopathy?

There is currently insufficient evidence that homeopathy is clearly efficacious for the treatment of any single clinical condition. Randomised trials have not been independently replicated for many of the conditions treated in homeopathic practice, such as depression, fatigue and eczema. However, many people have reported numerous benefits from homeopathy.

A recent study carried out by the NHS Centre for Reviews and Dissemination (based at York University) reviewed data from over 200 randomised clinical trials of homeopathy, but the data that did exist were of poor quality and came from trials that were often deeply flawed. Common problems included under-powered studies, failure to analyse by intention to treat and failure to use allocation concealment. Some of the published systematic reviews are criticised for pooling clinically heterogeneous data.

Despite many longstanding doubts, homeopathic remedies remain widely used in the NHS. There is insufficient evidence of the effectiveness of homeopathy either to recommend it as a treatment for any specific condition, or to warrant significant changes in the current provision of homeopathy (*Effective Health Care* 2002; **7**: 1–12). An analysis of trials of homoeopathy and conventional medicine estimated treatment effects in trials least likely to be affected by bias (*Lancet* 2005; **366**: 726–732). The results showed that biases are present in placebo-controlled trials of both homoeopathy and conventional medicine. When account was taken for these biases in the analysis, there was weak evidence for a specific effect of homoeopathic remedies, but strong evidence for specific effects of conventional interventions. This finding is compatible with the notion that the clinical effects of homoeopathy are placebo effects.

There are five homeopathic hospitals and it has been estimated that 20% of GP practices provide access to homeopathy (*BMJ* 2002; **324**: 565). Results of a small randomised controlled trial failed to show that homeopathic arnica had any advantage compared with placebo in reducing postoperative pain, bruising and swelling in patients having elective hand surgery (*J R Soc Med* 2003; **96**: 60).

Most trials of homeopathic medicines do not individualise treatment, which is obviously the hallmark of homeopathic practice. Moreover, randomisation and blinding of participants substantially distorts the context of homeopathic prescribing, thus potentially weakening its effect. There is much debate that a lack of supporting evidence does not mean these treatments are ineffective.

USEFUL WEBSITES

www.acupuncture.org.uk – British Acupuncture Council

www.bsmdh.org – British Society of Medical and Dental Hypnosis

www.osteopathy.org.uk – Osteopathic Information Service

www.mca.gov.uk – Medicines and Healthcare Products Regulatory Agency website

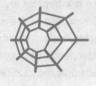

SUMMARY POINTS FOR COMPLEMENTARY MEDICINE

✓ The use of herbal medicines is increasing

✓ More research needs to be done regarding the efficacy of herbal medicines

✓ GPS should be aware of any herbal medicines their patients may be taking

✓ Many traditional Chinese medicines are harmful

CHAPTER 15:
MEDICOLEGAL ISSUES AND GUIDELINES

CHAPTER 15:
MEDICOLEGAL ISSUES AND GUIDELINES

General Medical Council

The General Medical Council (GMC) was established in 1858, and licenses doctors to practise in the UK under the provisions of the Medical Act 1983. The GMC's core functions are:

- ✓ Maintaining an up-to-date register of qualified doctors

- ✓ Fostering good medical practice

- ✓ Promoting high standards of medical education

- ✓ Protecting the public from doctors whose fitness to practise is in doubt.

The GMC produces a number of booklets setting out the standards which the Council expects individual doctors to follow. Of particular interest and relevance to general practice (and especially the MRCGP) are:

- ✓ *Good Medical Practice*

- ✓ *Confidentiality*

- ✓ *Consent: the Ethical and Legal Issues*

What is 'Good Medical Practice'?

In 1995 the GMC published a comprehensive statement (or code) setting out the principles of 'Good Medical Practice', at the core of which it listed the *'Duties of a Doctor'* – which should be read carefully, for the exam as well as for good clinical practice! *'Good Medical Practice'* now sets the framework of the professional standards within which doctors must practise in this country.

Doctors accepting GMC registration are therefore making a commitment to their patients and to their profession to practise accordingly. The GMC has recently set out a proposed third edition of *Good Medical Practice* with the intention of preparing doctors for revalidation checks.

What are the 'Duties of a Doctor'?

Doctors as a profession have a duty to maintain a good standard of practice and care and also show respect for human life. The guidelines emphasise what is expected of a doctor in practice today; they state a doctor must, among other things:

- ✓ Make the patients their first concern

- ✓ Treat patients politely and considerately and respect their dignity and privacy

- ✓ Listen to patients and respect their views

- ✓ Give patients information in a way they can understand

- ✓ Respect the rights of patients to be fully involved in decisions about their care

- ✓ Keep their professional knowledge and skills up to date

- ✓ Recognise the limits of their professional competence

- ✓ Be honest and trustworthy

- ✓ Respect and protect confidential information

- ✓ Make sure that their personal beliefs do not prejudice their patients' care

- ✓ Act quickly to protect patients from risk if the doctor has good reason to believe that himself or herself or a colleague may not be fit to practise

- ✓ Avoid abusing their position as a doctor

- ✓ Work with colleagues in the ways that best serve patients' interests.

In all these matters, doctors must never discriminate unfairly against their patients or colleagues and they must always be prepared to justify their actions to them.

USEFUL WEBSITE

www.gmc-uk.org – General Medical Council

SUMMARY POINTS FOR GENERAL MEDICAL COUNCIL

✓ GMC gives doctors licences to practise

✓ *Good Medical Practice* provides framework of professional standards

✓ Duties of a doctor are very important

Complaints

Complaints are a fact of life; the best approach is to manage them quickly and efficiently. Failure to satisfy a complainant at an early stage often results in the entrenchment of positions, and therefore ultimately demands a much greater investment of time in resolving the conflict. Complaints in general practice are increasing, and have been estimated to have increased threefold over the past 10 years. It is difficult to obtain exact figures because the majority of complaints are dealt with 'in-house' and so are only recorded in the practice records. The GMC guidance regarding complaints states that: 'Patients who complain about the care or treatment they have received have a right to expect a prompt, open, constructive and honest response. This will include an explanation of what has happened, and where appropriate, an apology. You must not allow a patient's complaint to prejudice the care or treatment you provide or arrange for that patient.'

What are common complaints in primary care?

The majority of complaints in primary care are dealt with promptly and efficiently, with minimal repercussions.

Common complaints include:

- ✓ Complications of requests for visits
- ✓ Prescribing errors
- ✓ Delay or missed diagnosis
- ✓ Delay in referral
- ✓ Failure to explain investigation or treatment plans
- ✓ Breach of confidentiality
- ✓ Failure to seek consent
- ✓ Unacceptable attitude on the part of professionals.

What is the complaints procedure?

The NHS patient complaints procedures have certain key objectives:

- ✓ Ease of access for patients and complainants
- ✓ A thorough and local resolution phase
- ✓ Fairness for both complainants and staff
- ✓ Investigation of complaints entirely separately from any subsequent disciplinary proceedings.

The process for dealing with complaints is relatively simple:

- ✓ The first stage is local resolution, to resolve the issue within the practice
- ✓ The second stage is an independent review
- ✓ The third stage is review by the Health Service Commissioner (Ombudsman) if requested by either the complainant or the doctor.

How are complaints dealt with in primary care?

All GPs are now required under the terms of service to operate a practice-based complaints procedure. A complaints manager should be appointed within each practice (usually the practice manager). The in-house procedure must be:

- ✓ Practice-owned and supported by all staff
- ✓ Adequately publicised with detailed written information.

When are complaints dealt with?

All complaints must:

- ✓ Be dealt with at the time, if a verbal complaint

- ✓ Be acknowledged within two working days

- ✓ Be given a full written response and explanation within 10 working days.

Complainants should always be invited to discuss the matter in an attempt to resolve it at an early stage.

SUMMARY POINTS FOR COMPLAINTS

- ✓ Complaints are common

- ✓ They should be resolved promptly

- ✓ Complaints procedure is simple to follow

- ✓ Most complaints are dealt with 'in-house'

Confidentiality

Confidentiality is both a legal and an ethical principle and is the cornerstone of medical practice. Confidentiality is, in theory, a very straightforward issue; however, translating it into practice often proves problematic. Confidentiality issues are far the commonest reason for doctors to contact medicolegal advisers for independent expert advice. Practitioners have a professional obligation to protect confidentiality and the presumption should always be made that all information is confidential. It is only under extreme circumstances (eg legal or moral duty) that confidentiality can be breached.

When can doctors disclose information without consent?

This question often crops up in the oral examination. Disclosure of personal information without consent, or against a patient's wishes, should only occur in the most exceptional circumstances; it may be justified when failure to do so may expose the patient or others to a risk of death or serious harm. Consent should be sought prior to disclosure where third parties are exposed to a risk so serious that it outweighs the patient's privacy interest. However, if this is not practicable, the information should be disclosed promptly to an appropriate person or authority.

This can occur in the following circumstances:

- ✓ Patient with an illness that is placing others at substantial risk (eg HIV infection)

- ✓ Patients continuing to drive against medical advice (see later)

- ✓ Where disclosure may assist in the prevention, detection or prosecution of a serious crime

- ✓ Death certificates

- ✓ Statutory requirement (eg the notification of communicable diseases)

- ✓ Following an order by a judge or presiding officer of a court

- ✓ When the patient is unable to give consent and it is in the patient's best interests (eg to relatives).

The GMC clearly states: 'Doctors who decide to disclose confidential information must be prepared to explain and justify their decision to the patient, if appropriate, and to the GMC and the courts, if called on to do so.'

Under which circumstances can doctors disclose information to the DVLA?

The Driver and Vehicle Licencing Agency (DVLA) is legally responsible for deciding if a person is medically unfit to drive, and patients have a legal duty to inform the DVLA of any medical condition that affects their ability to drive. The patient's doctor must make sure the patient understands that their medical condition may impair their ability to drive. If patients are incapable of understanding the advice (eg dementia) the DVLA must be informed immediately. If a patient refuses to inform the DVLA the doctor should make every reasonable effort to persuade the person to stop driving, which may even include telling the next of kin. If the patient cannot be persuaded to stop driving the doctor should then disclose the relevant medical information immediately, in confidence, to the medical advisor of the DVLA. Before giving the information to the DVLA, the patient should be informed of the doctor's decision to do so. Once the DVLA has been informed, a letter should be written to the patient confirming that the disclosure has been made.

SUMMARY POINTS FOR CONFIDENTIALITY

- ✓ Complaints are common
- ✓ Confidentiality must always be respected
- ✓ Should only be breached in extreme circumstances
- ✓ Data Protection Act has many implications

USEFUL WEBSITE

www.dvla.gov.uk – Medical standard of fitness to drive

Consent

Consent is a fundamental principle of medical law. Most doctors are aware of the importance of obtaining consent from their patients, but many are uncertain about what consent actually means and also fear that their instincts about what is right may not be enough to protect them from a legal challenge.

The case law on consent has evolved significantly over the past decade. The GMC has issued guidance on seeking patients' consent, which all registered practitioners in the UK should be aware of when counselling patients. For consent to be valid, three conditions must be satisfied.

First, the patient must be competent. Second, he or she must have sufficient information to make an informed choice; and, third, the consent must be given voluntarily.

Doctors must respect the right of their patients to be fully involved in decisions about their care. Wherever possible, they must be satisfied, before providing treatment or investigating a patient's condition, that:

- ✓ the patient has understood what is proposed and why; and understands any significant risks or side-effects associated with it

- ✓ has given consent.

Any competent adult has the right to give or withhold consent to an examination, investigation or treatment. Consent may be implied, oral or written. Consent should be based on information patients want to know and ought to know about their condition and treatment. This information should include:

- ✓ Details of the diagnosis and prognosis

- ✓ Results of undergoing treatment or refusing treatment

- ✓ Risks of uncertainties of treatment

- ✓ Possible complications of treatment.

Patients may change their mind and withdraw their consent at any time.

It should also be noted that no person can give consent for another adult; this is often not realised by many healthcare professionals.

What is meant by a 'competent adult'?

A competent adult must be able to:

- ✓ Understand the nature and purpose of treatment

- ✓ Understand the benefits, risks and alternatives

- ✓ Understand the consequences of refusal

- ✓ Retain the information long enough to make an effective decision

- ✓ Make a free choice.

Any mentally competent adult can refuse treatment for any reason (rational or irrational) or for no reason at all, even if doing so may result in his or her own death. In addition, a competent pregnant woman may refuse any treatment, even if it would be detrimental to the fetus.

What about consent for incompetent adults?

For an incompetent adult, the doctor should:

- ✓ Act in the patient's best interests

- ✓ Attempt to ascertain the patient's past wishes

- ✓ Review the medical and social knowledge of the patient's background, culture and religion

- ✓ Consult relatives, friends and carers

- ✓ Consider the option which least restricts the patient's future choices.

What about consent for children who lack capacity to consent?

Consent can be given on a child's behalf by any one person with parental responsibility or by the court. The Children Act 1989 describes who may have parental responsibility. These people include:

- ✓ The child's parents if they are married to each other at the time of conception or birth

- ✓ The child's mother (but not the father) if they were not so married, unless the father has acquired parental responsibility via a court order or a parental responsibility order or the couple subsequently marry

- ✓ The child's legally appointed guardian

- ✓ A person in whose favour the court has made a residence order

- ✓ A local authority designated in a care order of the child.

Failure to obtain a suitable consent may open a doctor to a GMC complaint, a civil claim or even criminal charges.

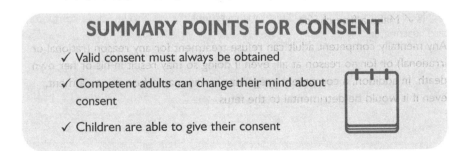

SUMMARY POINTS FOR CONSENT

- ✓ Valid consent must always be obtained

- ✓ Competent adults can change their mind about consent

- ✓ Children are able to give their consent

Medical negligence

It is widely known that the number of medical litigation cases continues to rise. To pursue a medical negligence claim a patient has to prove, on the balance of probability (ie meaning more likely than not), three things:

- ✓ The doctor owed a duty of care
- ✓ There was a breach of that duty
- ✓ Harm followed as a result.

What is the Bolam standard?

Independent medical doctors use the 'Bolam' standard to assess the doctor's clinical management. This means that the doctor has acted in a way that would be in agreement with a responsible body of doctors practising in the same field, and does not have to be the standard of the majority.

The Bolam test is another tenet of medical law which may be reviewed. This test defines the standard of care that doctors must meet, if they are not to be negligent. Patients' lawyers are keen to argue that it should not be a sufficient defence to a medical accident (especially when life is lost) to say that other responsible professionals would have done the same thing.

However, the courts have said they will depart from the professional practice approach if they see fit, the ultimate tests being what the court itself thinks was a reasonable amount of information to give the patient. This obviously leaves an element of doubt, as doctors cannot guess what the courts are going to say.

What is the commonest reason for a medical negligence claim?

A review of all claims involving GPs by the Medical Defence Union (MDU) found that almost half (45.5%) of all settled claims were related to a delay in a patient's diagnosis. However, a delay in diagnosis per se is not necessarily negligent, provided that the clinical management can be shown to be competent and reasonable.

However, the main problems are usually:

- ✓ Failure to examine properly

- ✓ Inadequate follow-up arrangements

- ✓ Lack of appropriate investigations

- ✓ Reports misfiled in the notes

- ✓ Poor communication with colleagues and patients

- ✓ Poor medical record keeping.

The increase in litigation in the UK does not reflect changing standards of clinical practice, which remains very high, but rather an increase in patients' expectations and their tendency to resort to litigation. The majority of claims do not go beyond disclosure of medical records, and less than 5% get as far as a court hearing.

SUMMARY POINTS FOR CONSENT

- ✓ Bolam standard often still used

- ✓ Most claims are due to delayed diagnosis

- ✓ Harm must result for a negligence claim

Guidelines

Clinical guidelines have increasingly become a familiar part of clinical practice. They have been defined as 'systematically developed statements to assist practitioner and patient decisions about appropriate healthcare for specific clinical circumstances.'

Clinical guidelines are only one option for improving the quality of care. They do, however, have both potential risks and harms. Guidelines should be practical, realistic and based on valid up-to-date evidence. They should also be easily accessible to practitioners, and should ideally be adapted to suit the local target population. They should always be practical and take into consideration the available resources needed for them to be successfully implemented.

The successful introduction of guidelines is dependent on many factors, including their clinical context and the methods used for developing, disseminating and implementing them. Ample evidence exists to support the argument that the most simple and cost-effective intervention to increase the implementation of guidelines is rewriting guidelines in behaviourally specific terms (*BMJ* 2004; **328**: 343).

Clinical guidelines are rarely based solely on research evidence; they often incorporate the consensus of experts.

Formal, structured methods for developing guidelines are used by NICE (*N Engl J Med* 2004; **351**: 1383). However, formal consensus methods often lack transparency and reliability; a new streamlined approach for producing guidelines has recently been proposed (*BMJ* 2005; **331**: 631).

What are NICE guidelines?

The National Institute for Clinical Excellence (NICE) was introduced in 1999 to appraise new technologies, including drugs, and decide which should be used in the NHS.

NICE was established to advise the NHS not only on the quality of care that individual patients could expect (in terms of appropriateness and effectiveness) but also to address the other important dimensions of healthcare quality (equity, fairness and efficiency) that society expects.

What are the problems with NICE?

One study assessed the extent and pattern of implementation of guidance issued by NICE (*BMJ* 2004; **329**: 999). It found that implementation was variable; some clinical practice has changed in line with NICE guidance, in particular around prescribing. Guidance seems to be more likely adopted when there is strong professional support and a stable and convincing evidence base, which is not the case for all of the NICE guidelines.

An analysis of some of the NICE guidelines by the *Drug and Therapeutics Bulletin* found that various guidelines, including those for influenza, type 2 diabetes and obesity, were unreliable.

One concern is that because all Primary Care Trusts (PCTs) are now compelled to implement NICE recommendations, the use of other effective treatments that have not yet been reviewed by the body may be cut, to contain costs. The NHS at a local level will probably have to dent other services' funding in order to fund NICE's recommendations. This will apply both to a specific intervention for which there is no NICE guidance and to whole services for which guidance is never likely (such as those for people with learning disabilities). By focusing on isolated, usually expensive new treatments, NICE is in danger of ignoring the wider picture; for example, in terms of improving quality of life for the elderly, demented patient, is it better to fund expensive medication or to improve the quality of nursing homes?

What are the benefits of guidelines?

✓ Improve the consistency of care

✓ Empower patients to make more informed choices

✓ Improve the quality of clinical decisions

✓ Can improve efficacy (save money)

✓ Reduce inappropriate practice.

What are the problems with guidelines?

✓ Recommendations may be wrong

✓ May be biased

✓ May be inflexible and not relate to individual patients

✓ Evidence used to write the guidelines is not always from appropriate, well-designed studies

✓ Can be time-consuming to use

✓ Need to be updated regularly

✓ Do not address all the uncertainties of clinical practice.

Another problem with guidelines is knowing which ones to use in clinical practice, as often different guidelines for the same condition have conflicting advice in them. This has recently been made apparent with the British Hypertension Society guidelines (*BMJ* 2004; **328**: 634). Although they recommend tailoring antihypertensive drug choice according to a patient's ethnic group and age (the ABCD approach), the NICE guidelines for hypertension state there is no evidence for this approach.

One study has demonstrated that most sets of guidelines do not modify or discuss their recommendations in older patients with co-morbidities (*JAMA* 2005; **294**: 716). Therefore, following clinical practice guidelines in the management of older patients with chronic diseases may be having a variety of unwanted effects.

What is the role of guidelines in court?

Guidelines could be introduced to a court by an expert witness as evidence of accepted and customary standards of care, but they cannot be introduced as a substitute for expert testimony. Courts are unlikely to adopt standards of care advocated in clinical guidelines as legal 'gold standards' because the mere fact that a guideline exists does not of itself establish that compliance with it is reasonable in the circumstances, or that non-compliance is negligent.

How easy is it to comply with guidelines?

One study has highlighted that it is not always easy to comply with guidelines, even if they are well-accepted guidelines. It showed that GPs targeted their actions regarding treatment for their patients with hypertension at a diastolic BP of 100 mmHg rather than at the recommended guideline of 90 mmHg, despite being aware of the guidelines (*Br J Gen Pract* 2001; **51**: 9–14).

Conversely, evaluation of clinical guidelines on the management of infertile couples has demonstrated that guidelines can lead to an improvement in GPs' performance (*BMJ* 2001; **322**: 1282–1284).

Guidelines are essentially written for the management of patient populations rather than for individuals. They will not address all the uncertainties of current clinical practice and should be seen as only one strategy that can help improve the quality of care that patients receive. Although guidelines are meant to tackle variations in practice there is always a risk of standardising practice around the average, which is not necessarily always the best for every clinical situation.

SUMMARY POINTS FOR GUIDELINES

✓ Guidelines should be easy to use

✓ Many conflicting guidelines exist

✓ Implementation of NICE guidelines is very variable

✓ Do not address all the uncertainties of clinical practice

CHAPTER 16:
ADVANCE DIRECTIVES AND END-OF-LIFE DECISIONS

CHAPTER 16: ADVANCE DIRECTIVES AND END-OF-LIFE DECISIONS

Advance directives

Definition

An advance directive gives patients the legal right to give or withhold consent to specific medical treatments in advance of becoming incompetent.

Since October 1999, people in England and Wales have been able to appoint a friend or relative to take healthcare decisions if they lose the ability to make their own decisions. This is termed a 'Continuing Power of Attorney' and allows the named person, called the 'proxy decision maker', to make decisions regarding the health and welfare of that person. Competence is best confirmed by having a person's signature witnessed by two people, one of whom should be a doctor capable of attesting to the person's state of mind.

BMA guidance regarding advance statements (living wills)

1. What is an advance statement?

People who understand the implications of their choices can state in advance how they wish to be treated if they suffer loss of capacity. An advance statement can be of various types:

✓ A requesting statement reflecting an individual's aspirations

✓ A statement of general beliefs and aspects of life which an individual values

✓ A statement that names another person who should be consulted at the time a decision has to be made

✓ A clear instruction refusing some or all medical procedures (advance directive)

✓ A statement which, rather than refusing any particular treatment, specifies a degree of irreversible deterioration after which no life sustaining treatment should be given

✓ A combination of the above, including requests, refusals and the nomination of a representative.

2. What form should an advance statement take?

An advance statement can be a written document, a witnessed oral statement, a signed printed card, a smart card or a note of a particular discussion recorded in the patient's file.

3. Who can make an advance statement?

Any person can make an advance statement including an individual under the age of 18.

4. Are advance statements legally binding?

A clear refusal of treatment by a competent adult, acting free from pressure, has potential legal force. General statements of preferences should be respected, but are not legally binding. Any advance statement is superseded by a clear and competent contemporaneous decision by the individual concerned.

5. Are all advance refusals of treatment legally binding?

An advance refusal is legally binding providing that the patient is an adult, the patient was competent and properly informed when reaching the decision, the statement is clearly applicable to the present circumstances and there is no reason to believe that the patient has changed his or her mind. If doubt exists about what the individual intended, the law supports a presumption in favour of providing clinically appropriate treatment, but where the situation that has arisen is clearly that which was envisaged by the patient, treatment should not be provided contrary to a valid advance refusal.

End-of-life decisions

✓ The Dutch have done most of the work in this field

✓ Doctors make end-of-life decisions in about 40% of deaths

✓ 75% involve withdrawing or withholding treatment.

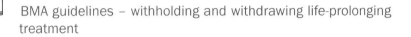

BMA guidelines – withholding and withdrawing life-prolonging treatment

Key principles

✓ Life cannot be preserved at all costs – treatment must be more of a benefit than a burden.

✓ Both artificial nutrition and hydration constitute medical treatment.

✓ Competent patients have the legal right to refuse treatment.

✓ Where patients cannot express their view doctors must take account of previously expressed wishes, the likelihood of any improvement and the likelihood of the patient experiencing severe pain or suffering.

✓ Close cooperation with the other professionals in the team is vital in decision-making.

✓ All proposals to withdraw or withhold artificial nutrition and hydration should be formally reviewed by a senior clinician who is not part of the team.

Withholding and withdrawing life-prolonging treatments: good practice in decision-making. London, GMC, 2002

The guidelines were prompted by concerns regarding the withdrawal of treatment from elderly patients and by inappropriate 'do not attempt resuscitation' orders. They set out the legal and ethical framework for taking decisions.

The guidelines remind doctors that patients who are mentally competent have a legal right to refuse treatment even if the outcome is certain death. Patients must not be assumed to lack mental capacity just because their decision might seem irrational or seems to doctors not to be in their best interests.

Doctors with a conscientious objection to a decision not to start or to continue with life-prolonging treatment may withdraw from the patient's care, but must hand the care over without delay to another suitably qualified colleague so that patient care does not suffer.

In Scotland, proxy decision-makers may be appointed for patients lacking the capacity to decide for themselves. However, in England and Wales, doctors must take decisions for patients who are mentally incompetent, acting in the patient's best interests and weighing up the benefits and burdens of the proposed treatment.

Doctors must not allow factors such as the patient's age, disability or lifestyle to prejudice the choice of treatment.

'Doctrine of double effect'

States that if measures taken to relieve physical or mental suffering cause the death of a patient, then it is morally and legally acceptable provided the doctor's intent is to relieve distress and not to kill the patient. In general, the doctor must make a full assessment of the patient's condition, consult with relatives, carers and other healthcare professionals involved in the case, and ask for a second medical opinion either from a specialist or from another GP.

1. Why active euthanasia and physician assisted suicide should be legalised (*BMJ* 2001; **323**: 1079–1080)

- ✓ Focused around the Dianne Pretty case (who suffered from motor neurone disease); the Court denied her the request of allowing her husband to aid her in ending her life.

- ✓ Argued that the moral and legal status of not saving a life through failing to treat can be the same as actively taking that life.

- ✓ Provided the circumstances are clinically warranted, doctors should be able to withdraw life-sustaining treatment when they intend to accelerate death as well as to relieve suffering.

2. Managing co-morbidities in patients at the end of life (*BMJ* 2004; **329**: 909–912)

This article highlighted the need for careful management in patients who develop a life-limiting illness. They outlined through case examples the difficulties that may arise and those areas that need special attention. In summary:

✓ Life-limiting illnesses include advanced cancer, end-stage organ failure, neurodegenerative disease, and AIDS.

✓ Both the life-limiting illness and co-morbidity change clinically over time and therefore need regular review.

✓ Decisions to adjust drugs should be taken actively as whole body changes occur in life-limiting illness, rather than based on adverse effects.

✓ Weight loss and other systemic changes reduce the need for many long-term drugs or alter their metabolism.

✓ Some long-term drugs should be continued until death while others should be ceased as systemic changes occur.

✓ Data on number needed to treat can be used to inform decisions about stopping long-term treatments.

CHAPTER 17:
MISCELLANEOUS
TOPICS

CHAPTER 17: MISCELLANEOUS TOPICS

Refugees

The issues regarding refugees, asylum-seekers and immigration have all been raised in the media over the last few years. There is a tendency to blame all of society's ills on asylum-seekers and laws on asylum are getting increasingly tough; for example, the controversial section 55 of the Nationality, Immigration and Asylum (NIA) Act of 2002 came into force on 8 January 2003 and denies asylum-seekers National Asylum Support Service (NASS) accommodation and financial benefits if they fail to apply for asylum as soon as reasonably practicable after their arrival in the UK. Potentially, this could mean destitution for many asylum-seekers arriving in the UK. Asylum-seekers affected by section 55 are still entitled to access primary or secondary healthcare services, and are eligible to apply for help with health costs (eg NHS prescriptions and dental care). In order to apply for help with health costs, an asylum-seeker must complete an HCI form, available from One Stop Services or the Health Benefits Division of the NHS. The issues of refugees are discussed in the summary below:

✓ The refugee population in Britain is highly diverse and is likely to remain large as conflicts continue to occur throughout the world.

✓ Refugees, unlike other migrants, have had to flee to escape oppression.

✓ The refugee population is concentrated in the Greater London area, but new legislation is resulting in dispersal throughout the UK.

✓ Refugees may be vulnerable to mental health problems, yet they have difficulty communicating their needs because of language barriers.

✓ All refugees, including asylum-seekers affected by section 55, are entitled to the full range of NHS services free of charge, including registration with a GP. The only exception is that, for asylum-seekers who have had their application rejected, hospitals have the right to decide on whether to charge, according to the 'individual's complete circumstances'.

✓ A strategic approach is needed to address the inequalities in primary care.

What happens to refugees?

✓ Refugee population is not evenly spread.

✓ Concentrated in areas where local authorities have given refugee housing a higher priority.

✓ Legislation will result in greater dispersal of refugees, making provision of specialist services more difficult.

✓ Part 2 of the NIA act outlines the setting up of 'accommodation centres' which should provide full-board accommodation, access to health services, education and training.

✓ 'Cultural bereavement' and coping with 'deeply disruptive change' are widely shared experiences of migration.

✓ Refugees are distinguished from other migrants by their lack of choice.

✓ Refugees have had to leave their countries of origin to escape persecution, imprisonment, torture or even death.

✓ Families may have been physically separated, causing much grief.

✓ Refugees are often preoccupied by worry about relatives left behind in their country of origin.

✓ Many refugees, including children, have no other relatives in the UK.

✓ Poverty and dissatisfaction with housing is widespread.

Health problems

✓ A recent UK study of Iraqi refugees found that all had been separated involuntarily from some close family members.

✓ 65% had a history of systematic torture during detention.

✓ 29% were unable to speak any English.

✓ Over 50% had significant psychological morbidity.

✓ Evidence that asylum-seekers who have not yet been granted the right to remain are under particular stress.

Deficiencies of primary care

✓ All refugees and asylum-seekers are entitled to the full range of NHS treatment free of charge.

✓ They have the right to register with a GP.

✓ There is evidence that some GPs are confused about this.

✓ Some patients are asked for their passports when trying to register, in fact GPs do not have the right to demand to see proof of identity.

✓ What happens to patients who are unable to produce a valid passport?

- Are they sent away?

- Who makes these decisions?

- Some practices are, perhaps reluctantly, open for refugees, whereas others are effectively closed, creating neighbouring general practices with very different demographic profiles and unequal needs

- When refugees join a GP's list they are often registered on a temporary rather than a permanent basis

- This removes financial incentives to undertake immunisation and cervical smear tests

- Why do GPs avoid giving refugees permanent registration status?

- High mobility of refugees is a myth – 70% of refugees had been living in their current home for more than a year (Home Office Survey 1995)

- Language barriers at the reception desk and in the consultation are common

- Health authorities lack interpreter services, generally not available outside working hours if they do exist

- Telephone interpreting using 'hands free' technology may offer a solution

- Lack of adequate professional interpreting services presents a barrier for all non-English-speaking patients, but this barrier is larger for those with psychological and emotional difficulties.

Increasing spending on refugee primary care

- ✓ Is fully justifiable on clinical and ethical grounds.

- ✓ Requires considerable political courage to prioritise refugees at a time when other groups in the population, such as elderly people and the mentally ill, have been identified as in need of more resources.

- ✓ It is important to remember that many refugees who settle in Britain have made valuable contributions to society.

What can be done to improve primary care for refugees?

- ✓ A strategic approach is required.

- ✓ Provide intensive courses in spoken English.

- ✓ The DoH needs to commission an information pack that includes a certificate of entitlement to NHS treatment and to develop patient-held medical records.

- ✓ The development of a national telephone interpreting service in a range of languages is a priority.

- ✓ A separate capitation payment for refugee patients, together with a new item of service payment linked to the duration of each professionally interpreted consultation, should be introduced.

- ✓ Healthcare facilitators should be recruited from each specific refugee population; they could help to provide patient-held records comprising an accurate and detailed medical history and to support health promotion and screening.

Conclusions

- ✓ The refugee population is likely to remain large.

- ✓ High needs, especially psychological distress, combined with language barriers require a great deal of additional time in consultations.

- ✓ GPs working in inner cities need adequate resources, especially interpreting services, and should be properly rewarded.

- ✓ A truly effective solution requires the political will to develop a comprehensive strategy at national level.

Recent advances in ethics

 1. Clinical review – Recent advances in medical ethics
(*BMJ* 2000; **321**: 282)

This interesting review focused on the continuing evolution of medical ethics through new technology, some of which could be envisaged making good viva material. The goal of medical ethics is to improve the quality of patient care by identifying, analysing and attempting to resolve the ethical problems that arise in practice.

Review advances in five areas:

1. End-of-life care

2. Medical error

3. Priority setting

4. Biotechnology

5. Medical ethics education

+ two future issues: 'eHealth' and 'global bioethics'.

1. End-of-life care

See Chapter 16.

2. Medical error

The main recent advance is the development of the Tavistock principles, which serve as an ethical foundation for those working to reduce medical error.

All the Tavistock principles are relevant to the problem of medical error, but the most important are:

✓ Cooperation with each other and those served is imperative for those working within the healthcare delivery system.

✓ All individuals and groups involved in healthcare, whether providing access or services, have the continuing responsibility to help improve its quality.

✓ In developing a culture of safety, clinicians will need to act as role models for their students by applying these principles themselves the next time they encounter a medical error.

✓ Healthcare leaders will need to 'feel personally responsible for error' and 'declare error reduction to be an explicit organisational goal and devote a significant proportion of the board and management agenda to achieving this goal'.

3. Priority setting

Development of an ethics framework – 'Accountability for Reasonableness' – for legitimate and fair decisions on setting priorities.

Priority setting = 'rationing' 20 years ago = 'resource allocation' 10 years ago and will be called 'sustainability' now.

The four conditions of 'Accountability for Reasonableness' are:

1. Publicity – decisions regarding coverage for new technologies (and other limit-setting decisions) and their rationales must be publicly accessible.

2. Relevance – these rationales must rest on evidence, reasons and principles that fair-minded parties (managers, clinicians, patients and consumers in general) can agree are relevant to deciding how to meet the diverse needs of a covered population under necessary resource constraints.

3. Appeals – there must be a mechanism for challenge and dispute resolution regarding limit-setting decisions, including the opportunity to revise decisions in the light of further evidence or arguments.

4. Enforcement – there must be either voluntary or public regulation of the process to ensure that the first three conditions are met.

4. Medical ethics education

✓ The revolution in information technology will dramatically change medical practice.

✓ Many ethical issues, including confidentiality of electronic medical records and the relationship of clinical records to research and management of health systems.

✓ Dramatic changes in the way doctors learn and access medical literature.

5.Global bioethics

✓ In this era of advanced globalisation the problems of medical ethics can no longer only be viewed from the perspective of wealthy countries.

✓ Global bioethics seeks to identify key ethical problems faced by the world's six billion inhabitants, and envisages solutions that transcend national borders and cultures.

✓ An International Association of Bioethics has been formed and a discussion board on global bioethics has been launched.

6. 'eHealth'

✓ The revolution in information technology will dramatically change medical practice.

✓ This raises many ethical issues, including how we can keep electronic medical records confidential and how we use our patient data to research and manage health systems.

✓ Doctors will also dramatically change the way they learn and access medical literature.

✓ A code of ethics for 'eHealth' has been developed by the internet.

✓ Healthcare Coalition are an organisation with representatives from industry, academic groups, government, patient and consumer organisations.

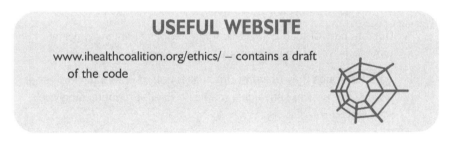

USEFUL WEBSITE

www.ihealthcoalition.org/ethics/ – contains a draft of the code

2. Editorial: Meeting the ethical needs of doctors (*BMJ* 2005; **330**: 741–742)

This interesting editorial champions the roles of ethicists in medicine; although aimed within hospital settings, it does highlight issues of potential relevance in general practice. Ethics remains poorly taught at undergraduate level, but is increasingly seen as core material on GP vocational training scheme (VTS) posts. In summary:

✓ A sound knowledge of medical ethics is essential to the good practice of medicine.

- ✓ Belief underlies the integration of medical ethics into the teaching of medical students.

- ✓ The BMA receives several thousand enquiries each year from concerned doctors confronted with ethical issues.

- ✓ Medical ethics is not only common sense.

- ✓ The emphasis in the teaching of medical ethics should be on identifying ethical problems, logical thinking, some knowledge of the relevant law and the importance of seeking help.

- ✓ Doctors may be unlikely to present their ethical concerns to a committee for fear of appearing foolish or ignorant.

- ✓ In North America, many hospitals have full time clinical ethicists as well as clinical ethics committees.

- ✓ Not all are from a medical background; most ethicists hold postgraduate degrees in subjects such as moral philosophy, theology, medical ethics and law, and they are increasingly trained in clinical ethics. May be on-call 24 h a day for staff or patients who need help in medico-ethical matters.

- ✓ Their task is to help resolve moral problems by drawing on their knowledge of ethical issues encountered in hospitals.

- ✓ Doctors may offload their ethical problems on clinical ethicists, abnegating their moral responsibilities too easily.

- ✓ Some sceptics may frown at the suggestion of creating yet another expert, but ethical cases, like medicine itself, are increasingly sophisticated.

- ✓ The author argues that we now need to introduce clinical ethicists in hospitals in the UK.

- ✓ Doctors cannot possibly deal with all the ethical problems they encounter in their professional lives, nor can they be expected to analyse complex ethical issues, and to know how similar cases were handled elsewhere. Clinical ethics committees cannot alone cope with the demands of ethically troubled doctors at the coalface.

- ✓ The use of clinical ethicists would represent an important step forward.

CHAPTER 18: THE CONSULTATION

CHAPTER 18:
THE
CONSULTATION

The next group of studies covers many areas of the consultation, at the end of which we will also look at recent studies of non-attendance and telephone consultations.

1. Deprivation, psychological distress, and consultation length in general practice (*Br J Gen Pract* 2001; **51**: 456–460)

Up to 40% of patients presenting to GPs are psychologically distressed, as measured by screening tools such as the General Health Questionnaire (GHQ). Of these distressed patients, doctors correctly identify about half. Poor mental health is a major predictor of future poor physical health. Failure to diagnose and treat appropriately may promote chronicity, inappropriate and unnecessary referral and medical treatment characteristic of somatic fixation. Correct identification of the patient's psychological problem may reduce somatisation. This study aimed to examine factors associated with the presentation and recognition of psychological distress in GPs' surgeries and the interaction of these factors with consultation length.

✓ This was a cross-sectional study involving 1075 consultations.

✓ The main outcome measures were patient psychological distress (measured by the GHQ), doctors' identification of psychological distress, consultation length and Carstairs Deprivation Category Scores.

✓ The results showed the mean consultation length was 8.71 min and the prevalence of positive GHQ scores was 44.7%. Increasing GHQ (greater psychological distress) and Lower Deprivation Category Scores (greater affluence) were associated with longer consultations.

✓ Positive GHQ scoring increased with greater socioeconomic deprivation and also peaked in the 30- to 39-year-old age group.

✓ Recognition of psychological distress was greater in longer consultations.

✓ They concluded that increasing socioeconomic deprivation is associated with a higher prevalence of psychological distress and shorter consultations.

✓ This provides further evidence to support Tudor Harts' 'inverse care law' (the availability of good-quality medical care is inversely proportional to its need) and has implications for the resourcing of primary care in deprived areas.

However, all the practices used in this study were involved in teaching and therefore potentially more motivated than average. Bias may also have resulted from participating GPs knowing that their 'performance' was being observed.

2. Patients' unvoiced agendas in general practice consultations: qualitative study (*BMJ* 2000; **320**: 1246–1250)

This qualitative study involved recording consultations and interviewing GPs the following day and the patients the following week. The results showed:

✓ Average of five points per patient agenda.

✓ Voiced agenda items were: most commonly symptoms, requests for diagnoses and prescriptions.

✓ Unvoiced agenda items were: worries about possible diagnosis, what the future holds, patients' ideas about what is wrong, side-effects, not wanting a prescription and information relating to social context.

✓ Only 4/35 patients voiced their full agendas.

✓ 24 patients voiced all their symptoms, but psychosocial issues were more likely not to be mentioned.

✓ Active steps should be taken in daily practice to encourage voicing of patients' agendas.

They concluded patients in primary care strongly want a patient-centred approach, with communication, partnership and health promotion. Improved communication can improve satisfaction and biomedical outcomes and involving patients in partnership can have benefits without increasing their anxiety. Patients with a very strong preference for patient centredness are those who are vulnerable either socioeconomically or because they are feeling particularly unwell or worried.

3. Observational study of effect of patient centredness and positive approach on outcomes of general practice consultations (*BMJ* 2001; **323**: 908–911)

This paper attempted to measure patients' perceptions of patient centredness and its relation to outcomes. It was an observational study using questionnaires involving 865 consecutive patients.

✓ Participants completed a short questionnaire before their consultation, in which they were asked to agree or disagree on a seven-point Likert scale with statements about what they wanted the doctor to do. A questionnaire after the consultation asked patients about their perception of the doctor's approach.

✓ Both questionnaires were based on the five main domains of the patient-centred model: exploring the disease and illness experience; understanding the whole person; finding common ground; health promotion; and enhancing the doctor–patient relationship.

✓ Patients were followed up after one month and the notes were reviewed after two months for re-attendance, investigation and referral.

✓ Main outcome measures were patients' enablement, satisfaction and burden of symptoms.

✓ Analysis identified five components:

- Communication and partnership (a sympathetic doctor interested in a patient's worries and expectations and who discusses and agrees the problem and treatment)

- Personal relationship (a doctor who knows the patient and their emotional needs)

- Health promotion

- Positive approach (being definite about the problem and when it would settle)

- Interest in effect on patient's life.

✓ Satisfaction was related to communication, partnership and a positive approach.

✓ Enablement was greater with interest in the effect on life, health promotion and a positive approach.

✓ A positive approach was also associated with reduced symptom burden at one month.

✓ Referrals were fewer if patients felt they had a personal relationship with their doctor.

The author concluded that 'if doctors don't provide a positive, patient centred approach patients will be less satisfied, less enabled, and may have greater symptom burden and higher rates of referral.'

4. An exploration of the value of the personal doctor–patient relationship in general practice (Br J Gen Pract 2001; 51: 712–718)

✓ Within the context of general practice, the opportunity exists for a personal relationship to develop between the patient and GP.

✓ This has benefits for both patients and GPs:

- Patient enablement is improved

- Compliance with medication is increased

- Clinical decision-making process and disclosure of psychosocial problems are facilitated

- The doctor–patient interaction itself can be therapeutic, enhanced by feelings of trust and understanding.

✓ The aims of this paper were to determine how many patients report having a personal doctor and when this is most valued, to compare the value of a personal doctor–patient relationship with that of convenience and to relate these findings to a range of patient, GP and practice variables.

✓ It was a cross-sectional postal questionnaire study involving 960 randomly selected adult patients.

✓ Qualitative interviews with patients and GPs were conducted and used to derive a parallel patient and GP questionnaire.

✓ The results showed that 75% of patients reported having at least one personal GP.

✓ The number of patients reporting a personal GP in each practice varied from 53% to 92%.

✓ Having a personal doctor–patient relationship was highly valued by patients and GPs, in particular for more serious psychological and family issues.

✓ 77–88% of patients and 80–98% of GPs valued a personal relationship more than a convenient appointment.

✓ For minor illness it had much less value.

They concluded that patients and GPs particularly value a personal doctor–patient relationship for more serious or for psychological problems. Whether a patient has a personal GP is associated with their perception of its importance and with factors that create an opportunity for a relationship to evolve.

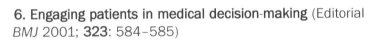

5. Long to short consultation ratio: a proxy measure of quality of care for general practice (*Br J Gen Pract* 1991; **41**: 48–54)

✓ Howie, in 1991, showed that longer consultations were linked to higher patient satisfaction.

✓ This was probably because the longer consultations dealt with more psychological and social issues.

6. Engaging patients in medical decision-making (Editorial *BMJ* 2001; **323**: 584–585)

✓ There is a consensus that patients ought to be more involved in their own care.

✓ Ethicists generally accept the principle that autonomy (what the competent, informed patient wants) trumps beneficence (what the doctor thinks best for the patient) in all but the most extreme circumstances.

✓ Quality in Health Care (September 2001) focused on engaging patients in medical decisions.

✓ 12 articles from an MRC conference. The proceedings gave a clear impression that although respecting patients' preferences is a fundamental goal of medicine, these preferences are vulnerable to manipulation and bias.

✓ Three questions dominated the debate:

1. Can patients take a leading role in making decisions?

2. Do they want to?

3. What if doctors and public health professionals don't like their choices?

In discussion of these:

✓ Decisions are complicated, and depend on patients' attitudes to risk.

✓ Some patients prefer a very bad outcome put off into the future to a moderately bad outcome occurring now.

✓ This is one of several reasons why patients' decisions are sometimes at odds with recommendations.

✓ Cultural beliefs can have a profound influence on decisions regarding treatment, eg some SE Asian cultures consider that surgery results in perpetual imbalance, causing the person to be physically incomplete in the next incarnation.

✓ May go some way to explain why fully informed, shared decision-making is so difficult to conduct in practice.

✓ Yet communication with patients can be improved, including evidence-based approaches such as training doctors, coaching patients and using aids to decision-making.

✓ However, not all patients want to make their own decisions. Yet there is a desire for information that is nearly universal.

The author concluded, 'Most patients want to see the road map, including alternative routes, even if they don't want to take over the wheel'.

7. Patient factors associated with duration of certified sickness absence and transition to long-term incapacity
(*Br J Gen Pract* 2004; **54**: 86–91)

This was a difficult study to categorise but was felt most relevant to how GPs consult and the effects that process can have on the patient. Despite a considerable increase in claims for long-term sickness benefits and the impact of certifying sickness upon GP workload, little is known about transition to long-term incapacity for work.

- ✓ The aim of the study was to explore the relationship between patient factors and the transition from short-term to long-term work incapacity, in particular focusing on mild mental health and musculoskeletal problems.

- ✓ Prospective data collection and audit of sickness certificate details.

- ✓ Claimant diagnosis, age, sex, postcode-derived deprivation score and sickness episode duration were all derived from the data collected.

- ✓ Mild mental disorder accounted for nearly 40% of certified sickness.

- ✓ Risk factors for longer-term incapacity included increasing age, social deprivation, mild and severe mental disorder, neoplasm and congenital illness.

- ✓ For mild mental disorder claimants, age, addiction and deprivation were risk factors for relatively longer incapacity.

- ✓ Back pain claimants were likely to return to work sooner than those with other musculoskeletal problems.

The authors concluded that, in addition to the presenting diagnosis, a range of factors is associated with the development of chronic incapacity for work, including age and social deprivation. GPs should consider these when negotiating sickness certification with patients. Although the study does not have any startling revelations it does confirm that sickness is multi-factorial and as GPs we should be aware that our actions carry many consequences.

8. Normalisation of unexplained symptoms by general practitioners: a functional typology (*Br J Gen Pract* 2004; **54**: 165–170)

Patients often present in primary care with physical symptoms that doctors cannot readily explain. The process of reassuring these patients is challenging, complex and poorly understood. The aim of this study was to construct a typology of GPs normalising explanations, based on their effect on the process and the outcome of consultations involving patients with medically unexplained symptoms.

- ✓ Qualitative analysis of audiotaped consultations between patients and GPs.

- ✓ Normalisation without explanation included rudimentary reassurance and the authority of a negative test result.

- ✓ Patients persisted in requesting explanation and elaborated or extended their symptoms, rendering somatic management more likely.

- ✓ Normalisation with ineffective explanation provided a tangible physical explanation for symptoms, unrelated to patient's expressed concerns. This was counterproductive.

- ✓ Normalisation with effective explanation provided tangible mechanisms grounded in patients' concerns, often linking physical and psychological factors. These explanations were accepted by patients; those linking physical and psychological factors contributed to psychosocial management outcomes.

- ✓ The routine exercise of normalisation by GPs contains approaches that are ineffective and may exacerbate patients' presentation. However, it also contains types of explanation that may reduce the need for symptomatic investigation or treatment.

These findings can inform the development of well-grounded educational interventions for GPs.

9. Eliciting patients' concerns: a randomised controlled trial of different approaches by the doctor (*Br J Gen Pract* 2004; **54**: 663–666)

Although a 'patient-centred' approach to general practice consultation is widely advocated, there is mixed evidence of its benefits.

- ✓ The aim of the RCT was to measure the costs and benefits of using a prompt to elicit patients' concerns when they consult for minor illness.

- ✓ Patients identified during the first part of the consultation as having a self-limiting illness were randomised to a second part of the consultation that was conducted 'as usual' or involved a written prompt to elicit the patient's concerns.

- ✓ After each consultation the doctor noted the diagnosis and the consultation length and the patient self-completed a questionnaire containing measures of satisfaction, enablement and anxiety.

- ✓ Patients in the elicitation group reported a small but significant increase in the 'professional care' score of the consultation satisfaction questionnaire but no other benefits were detected.

- ✓ Consultations in the elicitation group, however, were longer by about a minute.

- ✓ They concluded given the pressures on consultation time in general practice that there must be questions about the practical value of eliciting patients' concerns if the benefit of doing so is small and the cost large.

A controversial conclusion when this forms a cornerstone of consultation skills within general practice education; it will be interesting to see if any further studies are done for other parts of the consultation.

10. Shared decision making and risk communication in practice: a qualitative study of GPs' experiences *(Br J Gen Pract* 2005; **55**: 6–13)

Important barriers to the wider implementation of shared decision-making remain. The experiences of professionals who are skilled in this approach may identify how to overcome these barriers.

- ✓ The aims of this qualitative study were to identify the experiences and views of professionals skilled in shared decision-making and risk communication, exploring the opportunities and challenges for implementation.

- ✓ Interventions comprised training in shared decision-making skills and the use of risk-communication materials.

- ✓ The GPs indicated positive attitudes towards involving patients and described positive effects on their consultations.

- ✓ However, the frequency of applying the new skills and tools was limited outside the trial. Doctors were selective about when they felt greater patient involvement was appropriate and feasible, rather than seeking to apply the approaches to the majority of consultations. They felt they often responded to consumer preferences for low levels of involvement in decision-making.

- ✓ Time limitations were important in not implementing the approach more widely.

They concluded the promotion of 'patient involvement' appears likely to continue. Professionals appear receptive to this, and willing to acquire the relevant skills.

Strategies for wider implementation of patient involvement could address how consultations are scheduled in primary care, and raise consumers' expectations or desires for involvement.

11. Chaperones for intimate examinations: cross sectional survey of attitudes and practices of general practitioners (*BMJ* 2005; **330**: 234–235)

The conduct of intimate examinations in medical settings has been a subject of controversy for many years, because of potential difficulties and pitfalls for both doctors and patients.

The use of chaperones by male doctors has substantially increased over the past 20 years, with a continuing low level of use by female doctors, despite one-third of practices having a policy. Record keeping about the offer and use of chaperones is poor, and significant barriers to the use of appropriate chaperones in general practice still undoubtedly exist. The recommendations of the royal colleges and other bodies are, therefore, difficult to implement fully.

Some studies have shown, however, that the attitudes and behaviour of medical professionals are often at odds with recommendations and that patients may not always welcome the offer, let alone the presence, of a third person in the consultation.

They describe the attitudes and practices of general practitioners regarding the involvement of chaperones during intimate examinations and identify barriers and concerns affecting their use.

✓ A self completion questionnaire, with 38 items, was developed from themes emerging from patient focus groups and was piloted and modified before being sent to 1813 doctors from 18 primary care trusts in England, selected to achieve geographical and demographic diversity.

✓ The mean age of respondents was 45 (range 27–69); 754 (61%) were male and 972 (78%) were white. In all, 890 practices (71%) were urban, with 132 (11%) rural and 203 (16%) intermediate. There were more female GPs in rural practices and more GPs from ethnic minorities in urban practices.

✓ A total of 37% respondents had a policy on the use of chaperones.

✓ Altogether 68% of male GPs and 5% of female GPs usually or always offered a chaperone.

✓ 410 (54%) men and 9 (2%) women usually or always used a chaperone.

✓ 60 males (8%) and 344 females (70%) never used one.

✓ Use of chaperones was correlated with increasing age, belonging to a non-white ethnic group and working in a smaller practice.

✓ Practice nurses were the most common chaperones.

✓ A family member or accompanying person (47%), a non-clinical member of the practice staff (43%), a student or GP registrar (22%) or another doctor (10%) were alternatives. Most respondents rarely or never recorded the offer (66%) or the identity (71%) of a chaperone.

The authors conclude that more flexible guidance is needed for general practice, which must recognise the realities of current staffing and space arrangements, and take greater account of the wider context of the relationship between patients, their doctors and the practice. Further research is needed into patients' views and wishes.

12. Editorial: Clinical and communication skills need to be learnt side by side (*BMJ* 2005; **330**: 374–375)

When working with patients and colleagues, communication and clinical skills are practised simultaneously, yet most medical school curriculums teach them separately, albeit in parallel.

✓ The current practice of teaching communication skills separately from clinical skills reflects a reductionist paradigm – by breaking down the complex phenomenon of a consultation to its basic components. This may be helpful at an early stage of learning, but it may limit the coherence needed to ensure that doctors communicate satisfactorily with patients.

✓ In the United Kingdom and United States, the divergence has been compounded by evidence that most complaints are related to poor communication.

✓ This has led to a greater emphasis on communication skills. The increasing predominance of early community-based learning where communication skills are emphasised has also contributed to this dichotomy.

✓ Teaching communication and clinical skills separately does not mirror clinical experience and may lead to unbalanced doctors.

✓ Clinicians with sound clinical knowledge may be appraised of the latest research evidence yet unable to translate their skills into effective clinical care.

✓ Poor communication can often lead to poor health management.

✓ Learning communication and clinical skills side by side would address how important skills for clinical practice can be improved.

✓ Evidence from RCTs shows that interactive continuing medical education is effective in changing clinical performance.

Non-attendance

Non-attendance at general practices and outpatient clinics. Local systems are needed to address local problem (*BMJ* 2001; **323**: 1081–1082)

This editorial looked at the problem of non-attendance, the ramifications and thoughts regarding solutions.

At times of increasing debate on rationing of resources, this topic tends to be increasingly mentioned in the medical press.

In summary

✓ Non-attendance at NHS outpatient clinics and at general practices is more common in deprived populations.

✓ The national figure of 12% for non-attendance at outpatient clinics in the UK hides large variations between specialties and between regions.

✓ Much less research has been done on non-attendance in general practices, though figures of 3% and 6.5% have been reported.

✓ Non-attendance in general practices are associated with youth and deprivation, but not sex.

✓ Non-attenders are less likely to own a car or a telephone and are more likely to be unemployed.

✓ Some non-attendance arises from an inability to cancel the appointment, either because the hospital's system for cancelling or changing appointments is poor or because the patient has no access to a telephone.

✓ Non-attendance is not thought to be related to the severity of the patient's condition, except in the case of psychiatric illness where non-attendance may be a marker of severity of illness.

✓ The commonest reasons cited for missing an appointment, after forgetting it, are family or work commitments.

✓ Patients with lower paid jobs may have difficulty in getting time off work or arranging childcare.

✓ These reasons also partly explain the peak age range of 20–30 years in non-attenders, as this is the usual age for raising a family.

✓ The key seems to be to allow the patient to select a suitable time and date; indeed, such flexibility may largely explain the lower non-attendance rate in general practices, although evening surgeries and shorter time intervals to the appointment probably also contribute.

✓ The strongest predictor of non-attendance is the time interval to the appointment; reducing non-attendance reduces waiting times, which further reduces non-attendance, creating a virtuous circle.

✓ Increased consumerism in the NHS means that current systems are stale, at best.

✓ No single solution will work across the NHS and in outpatient clinics as well as general practices.

✓ Local trusts in primary and secondary care should be able to devise local systems to allow convenient access for their patients.

✓ New systems should be the subject of research and development.

✓ Non-attendance should fall if some of these measures are adopted, though it will never disappear – we are all human!

Telephone consultations

Telephone consultations to manage requests for same-day appointments: a randomised controlled trial in two practices
(*Br J Gen Pract* 2002; **52**: 306–310)

GPs in the UK have recently begun to adopt the use of telephone consultation during daytime surgery as a means of managing demand, particularly requests for same-day appointments. However, it is not known whether the strategy actually reduces GP workload.

✓ The aim of this study was to investigate how the use of telephone consultations impacts on the management of requests for same-day appointments, on resource use, indicators of clinical care and patient perceptions of consultations.

✓ It was an RCT of all patients (*n*=388) seeking same-day appointments in each surgery in two urban practices (total population 10,420) over a 4-week period.

✓ The primary outcome measure was use of doctor time for the index telephone or face-to-face consultation.

✓ Secondary outcomes were subsequent use of investigations and of services in the 2-week period following consultation, frequency of blood pressure measurement and antibiotic prescriptions and number of problems considered at consultation.

✓ Patient perceptions were measured by the Patient Enablement Instrument (PEI) and reported willingness to use telephone consultations in the future.

✓ The results showed telephone consultations took less time (8.2 vs 6.7 min).

✓ Patients consulting by telephone re-consulted the GP more frequently in the 2 weeks that followed.

✓ There was no significant difference in patient perceptions or other secondary outcomes.

The authors concluded that the use of telephone consultations for same-day appointments was associated with time-saving, and did not result in lower PEI scores. Possibly, however, this short-term saving was offset by a higher re-consultation rate and less use of opportunistic health promotion.

Consultation models

During my registrar year, it seemed a trivial task to learn consultation models in order to pass the exam and show some knowledge when asked. However, I have come to realise that learning these models is one step closer to an increased awareness of how your consultations work, that they are of benefit in predicting outcome and that as time passes they become second nature.

My argument is that, despite the endless debate of increased paperwork taking time away from patient contact and increased managerial responsibilities, the core of your daily routine remains a one-to-one patient interaction. If this can be achieved more efficiently, with greater satisfaction for the patient leading to less re-attendance, you would expect there to be an endless line of takers. However, that is not the case. The techniques are often forgotten shortly after the registrar year has ended, and rarely does one look back. As food for thought for those of you who remain free of too much cynicism, these models and their various facets do work in allowing less stressful and more fruitful consultations. They can help you with your stress levels and ultimately keep you going. Use them and experiment during the trainee year, and after if you are so inclined; everybody's style is different and you may find some facets too difficult or unproductive. Obviously you will concentrate on getting your video done, but this still allows tuning of your consultation. For those of you lucky few who were genuinely inspired by your trainer, remember it takes years of practice to make slick consultations look easy, but it is attainable – just enjoy getting there.

For those of you taking the exam, it is advisable to learn the models and some working clinical case models to illustrate certain points. This may be a question in your viva and certainly there is always an odd MCQ or two.

Biomedical model

The classic medical diagnostic process

- ✓ Observation: history and examination
- ✓ Hypothesis: provisional diagnosis
- ✓ Hypothesis testing: investigations
- ✓ Deduction: definitive diagnosis.

In essence, this is a hypothetico-deductive model but:

- ✓ Reductionist: patient is regarded as a collection of signs, symptoms and diagnosis.

- ✓ Doctor-centred; patient's ideas, concerns and expectations ignored.

- ✓ Sharing information not important. Emphasis not placed on agreeing management plan.

- ✓ No progress can be made if no objective physical disorder is unearthed.

- ✓ Omits use of doctor–patient relationship.

Other models have been developed that are more holistic:

- ✓ Not competing, but complementary.

- ✓ Several are often needed to give a broad understanding of something as complex as human interaction.

Alternative models

Byrne and Long Phase I

- ✓ Phase I: the doctor establishes a relationship with the patient.

- ✓ Phase II: the doctor either attempts to discover or actually discovers the reason for the patient's attendance.

- ✓ Phase III: the doctor conducts a verbal or physical examination, or both.

- ✓ Phase IV: the doctor, or the doctor and the patient, or the patient (in that order of probability) considers the condition.

- ✓ Phase V: the doctor, and occasionally the patient, details further treatment or further investigation.

- ✓ Phase VI: the consultation is terminated, usually by the doctor.

Used the terms 'Doctor-centred' and 'Patient-centred'. This model was produced after analysing more than 2000 tape recordings of consultations.

Pendleton, Schofield, Tate and Havelock

Seven tasks:

1. To define the reason for the patient's attendance, including: the nature and history of the problems; their aetiology; the patients' ideas, concerns and expectations; the effects of the problems.

2. To consider other problems: continuing problems and risk factors.

3. With the patient, to choose an appropriate action for each problem.

4. To achieve a shared understanding of the problems with the patient.

5. To involve the patient in the management and encourage him or her to accept responsibility.

6. To use time and resources appropriately: in the consultation and in the long term.

7. To establish or maintain a relationship with the patient which helps to achieve the other tasks.

Emphasises both the importance of the patient's view and understanding of the problem. Includes the term 'Consultation mapping.'

Stott and Davis

- ✓ Management of presenting problems.

- ✓ Modification of help-seeking behaviour.

- ✓ Management of continuing problems.

- ✓ Opportunistic health promotion.

Neighbour

- ✓ The inner consultation.

- ✓ Connecting: needs rapport-building skills.

- ✓ Summarising: needs listening and eliciting skills to facilitate effective assessment.

- ✓ Hand over: needs communicating skills to hand over responsibility for management.

✓ Safety netting: needs predicting skills to suggest contingency plan for worst scenario.

✓ Housekeeping: needs self-awareness to clear your mind of the psychological remains of one consultation so that it has no detrimental effect on the next (clearing your head).

Rosenstock, Becker and Maiman

Health beliefs' model

It shows the patient is more likely to accept advice, diagnosis or treatment if the doctor is aware of their ideas, concerns and expectations.

Patient's behaviour is determined by:

✓ Alarming symptoms.

✓ Trigger factors such as advice from family and friends, messages from media.

✓ Health motivation (interest in health).

✓ Perceived vulnerability to the condition.

✓ Perceived seriousness of the condition.

✓ Perceived balance of benefits of treatment against costs.

✓ Belief that the doctor has/has not understood the patient's concerns.

Heron

Six-category intervention model

Doctor can use any of six types of intervention:

1. Prescriptive: instructions; advice.

2. Informative: explanations; interpretations; new knowledge.

3. Confronting: feedback on behaviour; challenging but caring attitude.

4. Cathartic: aiding release of emotions in form of anger, laughter, crying.

5. Catalytic: encouraging patient to explore feelings, thoughts and behaviour.

6. Supportive: bolstering self-worth.

Berne

Transactional analysis ('games people play')

Explores behaviour within relationships. Identifies three 'ego-states':

- ✓ Parent: critical or caring

- ✓ Adult: logical

- ✓ Child: spontaneous or dependent.

Examines implications of, and reasons for, the different states. Explores 'games' – useful for analysing why consultations repeatedly go wrong and encouraging doctors to break out of these unproductive cycles of behaviour.

Balint

 The doctor, his patient and the illness (1957) (New York, Balint. International University Press)

The doctor–patient relationship is fundamental. Patients are more than broken machines, and doctors have feelings, which have a function in the consultation.

Proposed:

- ✓ Psychological problems are often manifested physically and even physical disease has its own psychological consequences which need particular attention.

- ✓ Doctors have feelings and those feelings have a function in the consultation.

- ✓ There needs to be specific training to produce limited but considerable change in the doctor's personality so that he or she can become more sensitive to the patient's thoughts during the consultation.

The doctor must:

- ✓ Discover the patient's beliefs, concerns and expectations about the problem or problems presented.

- ✓ Share his/her own understanding of the problems with the patient in terms that are understood by the patient.

✓ Share the decision-making with the patient.

✓ Encourage the patient to take appropriate responsibility for his/her own health.

KEY CONCEPTS AND PHRASES

1. The doctor as a drug

2.   The child as the presenting complaint:

   ✓ Patient may offer another person (eg child) as the problem when there are underlying psychosocial problems

3. Elimination by appropriate physical examination

   ✓ May reinforce the patient's belief that neurotic symptoms are in fact due to physical illness

4. Collusion of anonymity:

   ✓ Mistaken beliefs in the origin of symptoms are reinforced by examination

   ✓ Responsibility of uncovering underlying problems becomes increasingly diluted by repeated referral

   ✓ No-one takes responsibility

5. The mutual investment company:

   ✓ Formed and managed by the doctor and the patient

   ✓ 'Clinical illnesses' equal 'Offers' in a long relationship

   ✓ 'Offers' of problems (physical and psychosocial) are presented to the doctor for his 'Acceptance'

6. The flash:

   ✓ When the real reason of the 'Offer' (underlying psychosocial and neurotic illness) is suddenly apparent to both doctor and patient

   ✓ Acts as a central point for change

   ✓ Consultation can now deal with the underlying basic 'Fault'

Note

For the exam, think of clinical scenarios to illustrate each of the above and understand what is meant by each term.

Triaxial model

Address patient's problem in:

1. Physical terms

2. Psychological terms

3. Social terms.

 Tate's tasks From The Doctors' Communication Handbook

Involves the use of concepts featured in other models. Similar to those used to assess tasks in the summative assessment and MRCGP videos.

1. Discover the reasons for attendance:

    • Listen to the patient's description of the symptom

    • Obtain relevant social and occupational information

    • Explore the patient's health understanding

    • Enquire about other problems

    • Obtain additional information about critical symptoms or other details

    • Appropriate physical examination

    • Make a working diagnosis

2. Define the clinical problem(s):

    • Address the patient's problem(s)

    • Assess the severity of the presenting problem

    • Choose an appropriate form of management

    • Involve the patient in the management plan to the appropriate extent

3. Explain the problem(s) to the patient:

- Share your findings with the patient

- Tailor the explanation to the needs of the patient

- Ensure that the explanation is understood and accepted by the patient

4. Make effective use of the consultation:

- Make efficient use of resources – time, investigations, other professionals, etc

- Establish an effective relationship with the patient.

Glossary

AA	Alcoholics Anonymous
ACE	angiotensin-converting enzyme; also Asthma Control and Expectations
ACEI	angiotensin-converting enzyme inhibitor
ACS	Acute coronary syndrome
AD	Alzheimer's disease
ADFAM National	National Charity for the Families and Friends of Drug Misusers
ADHD	attention deficit-hyperactive disorder
AF	atrial fibrillation
AIDS	acquired immunodeficiency syndrome
AOM	acute otitis media
ARB	angiotensin-II receptor blocker
ARR	Absolute risk reduction
b	billion (1,000,000,000)
BHS	British Hypertension Society
BMA	British Medical Association
BMD	bone mineral density
BMI	body mass index
BNF	British National Formulary
BNP	B-type natriuretic peptide
BP	blood pressure
BPH	Benign prostatic hyperplasia
BTS	British Thoracic Society
CAMS	Cannabis in Multiple Sclerosis [trial]
CAP	Comparison Arm for ProtecT
CARDS	Collaborative AtoRvastatin Diabetes Study
CBT	cognitive behaviour therapy
CFC	chlorofluorocarbon
CG	clinical governance
CHARM	Candesartan in Heart Failure Assessment of Reduction in Mortality and Morbidity
CHD	coronary heart disease
CHF	Chronic heart failure

CHI	Commission for Health Improvement
CIBIS	Cardiac Insufficiency Bisoprolol Study
CNS	Central nervous system
COAD	chronic obstructive airways disease
COCP	combined oral contraceptive pill
COMET	Carveilol or Metoprolol European Trial
COPD	Chronic Obstructive Pulmonary Disease
CPA	care programme approach
CPD	continuous professional development
CPR	cardiopulmonary resuscitation
CRHP	Council for the Regulation of Healthcare Professionals
CSM	Committee on the safety of medicine
CT	computed tomography
CVA	cardiovascular accident
CVD	cardiovascular disease
CXR	Chest x-ray
DBP	diastolic blood pressure
DC	Direct current
DCCT	Diabetes Control and Complications Trial
DEXA	dual-energy X-ray absorptiometry
DHA	Docasahexaenoic acid
DICS	Ductal carcinoma in situ
DNR	do not resuscitate
DoH	Department of Health
DSH	Deliberate self-harm
DTI	Department of Trade and Industry
DVLA	Driver and Vehicle Licencing Agency
DVT	deep vein thrombosis
EBM	evidence-based medicine
ECG	Electrocardiogram
EHC	Emergency hormonal contraception
EPA	Eicosapentaenoic acid
EU	European Union
FOBT	Faecal occult blood test
GHQ	General Health Questionnaire
GMC	General Medical Council
GMS	General Medical Services
GP	general practitioner

GPC	General Practitioners' Committee
GUM	genitourinary medicine
HA	health authority
Hb	Haemoglobin
HDL	high-density lipoprotein
HIV	human immunodeficiency virus
HMP	Her Majesty's Prisons
HON	Health on the Net
HOPE	Healthcare Options Plan Entitlement
HOT	Hypertension Optimal Treatment [trial]
HPS	Heart Protection Society
HRT	hormone replacement therapy
IAG	Independent advisory group
IC	independent contractor
IGT	Impaired glucose intolerance
IHD	ischaemic heart disease
IUCD	intrauterine contraceptive device
LABA	Long-acting beta-2-agonist
LARC	Long-acting reversible contraception
LBC	Liquid-based cytology
LCR	ligase chain reaction
LDL	low-density lipoprotein
LIFT	Local Improvement Finance Trust
LRTI	lower respiratory tract illness
LTRAs	Leukotriene receptor antagonists
LVD	Left ventricular dysfunction
LVH	left ventricular hypertrophy
m	million
MDU	Medical Defence Union
MERIT-HF	Metoprolol CR/XL Randomised Intervention Trial in Congestive Heart Failure
MI	myocardial infarction
MMR	measles, mumps and rubella
MMSE	Mini-Mental State Examination
MMT	methodone maintenance treatment
MND	motor neurone disease
MRC	Medical Research Council
MS	multiple sclerosis

MWS	Million women study
NAAT	Nucleic acid amplification technology
NASS	National Asylum Support Service
NCAA	National Clinical Assessment Authority
NCSP	National Chlamydia screening programme
NeLH	The National electronic Library for Health
NI	National Insurance
NIA	Nationality, Immigration and Asylum Act
NICE	National Institute for Clinical Excellence
NMDA	N-methyl-D-aspartate
NNT	number needed to treat
NPFIT	National Programme for Information Technology
NRT	nicotine replacement therapy
NSAID	Non-steroidal anti-inflammatory drugs
NSF	National Service Framework
OA	osteoarthritis
OGTT	oral glucose tolerance test
PAAPs	Personal asthma action plans
PAD	Peripheral arterial disease
PBC	Practice-based commissioning
PBR	Payment by results
PCG	primary care group
PCOs	Primary Care Organisation
PCT	primary care trust
PD	Parkinson's Disease
PE	pulmonary embolism
PEFR	Peak expiratory flow rate
PEI	Patient Enablement Instrument
PFI	Private Financial Initiatives
PHCT	primary healthcare team
PID	Pelvic inflammatory disease
PMS	personal medical services
POP	Progesterone only pill
PPDPs	Practice and Personal Development Plan
PROGRESS	Peridopril pROtection aGainst REcurrent Stroke Study
ProtecT	Prostate testing for cancer and Treatment
PSA	prostate-specific antigen
PTSD	Post traumatic stress disorder

PVD	Peripheral vascular disease
QMAS	Quality management and analysis system
QOF	Quality and outcome framework
RCGP	Royal College of General Practioners
RCN	Royal College of Nursing
RCOG	Royal College of Obstetricians and Gynaecologists
RCP	Royal College of Physicians
RCPsych	Royal College of Psychiatrists
RCT	randomised controlled trials
SBP	systolic blood pressure
SERMs	selective oestrogen-receptor modulators
SMAC	Standing Medical Advisory Committee
SMAS	Substance Misuse Advisory Service
SPAF	Stroke Prevention in Atrial Fibrillation [trial]
SSRI	selective serotonin-reuptake inhibitors
STD	sexually transmitted disease
STI	sexually transmitted infection
STORM	Sibutramine Trial of Obesity Reduction and Maintenance
TC	total cholesterol
TCA	tricyclic antidepressant
TIA	transient ischaemic attack
TNT	Treating to New Targets
TSH	Thyroid-stimulating hormone
UKPDS	UK Prospective Diabetes Study
ValHeFT	Valsartan Heart Failure Trial
VTE	venous thromboembolism
VTS	Vocational Training Scheme
WHI	Women's Health Initiative [study]
WHO	World Health Organisation
WOSCOPS	West of Scotland Coronary Prevention Study

Journals referenced in this book

Alcohol Alcoholism	Alcohol Alcoholism
Am J Cardiol	American Journal of Cardiology
Am J Med	American Journal of Medicine
Ann Int Med	Annals of Internal Medicine
Arch Intern Med	Archives of International Medicine
Arch Neurol	Archives of Neurology
Asthma	Asthma
BJGP	British Journal of General Practice
BJU	British Journal of Urology
BJU Int	BJU (British Journal of Urology) International
BMJ	British Medical Journal
Br J Cancer	British Journal of Cancer
Br J Cardiol	British Journal of Cardiology
Br J Clin Pharmacol	British Journal of Clinical Pharmacology
Br J Diabetes Vasc Dis	British Journal of Diabetes and Vascular Disease
Br J Ophthalmol	British Journal of Ophthalmology
Br J Psychiatry	British Journal of Psychiatry
Can Med Assoc J	Canadian Medical Association Journal
Circulation	Circulation
Clin Evid	Clinical Evidence
Cochrane Library	Cochrane Library
Contraception	Contraception
Current Med Res Opin	Current Medical Research and Opinion
Diabetes	Diabetes
Diabetes Care	Diabetes Care
Diabet Primary Care	Diabetes and Primary Care
Diabetes Res Clin Practice	Diabetes Research and Clinical Practice
Drug Ther Bull	Drug and Therapeutics Bulletin
Effective Healthcare	Effective Healthcare
Emerg Med J	Emergency Medicine Journal
Eur Heart J	European Heart Journal

Eur J Clin Pharmacology	European Journal of Clinical Pharmacology
Eur Respir J	European Respiratory Journal
Family Practice	Family Practice
Gynecol	Gynecology
Health Promot Int	Health Promotion International
Hypertension	Hypertension
Int J Clin Pract	International Journal of Clinical Practice
Int J Ger Psychiatry	International Journal of Geriatric Psychiatry
J Am Geriatr Soc	Journal of the American Geriatrics Society
J Bone Miner Res	Journal of Bone and Mineral Research
J Card Fail	Journal of Cardiac Failure
J Child Psychol	Journal of Child Psychology
J Clin Endocrinol Metab	Journal of Clinical Endocrinology and Metabolism
J Clin Epidemiol	Journal of Clinical Epidemiology
J Consult Clin Psychol	Journal of Consulting and Clinical Psychology
J Fam Pract	Journal of Family Practice
J Gen Intern Med	Journal of General Internal Medicine
J Hum Hypertens	Journal of Human Hypertension
J Int Med Res	Journal of International Medical Research
J Med Screening	Journal of Medical Screening
J Natl Cancer Inst	Journal of the National Cancer Institute
J Paediatr Adolesc	Journal of Paediatrics and Adolescent Medicine
J Public Health Med	Journal of Public Health Medicine
J R Soc Med	Journal of the Royal Society of Medicine
JAMA	Journal of the American Medical Association
Lancet	Lancet
N Engl J Med	New England Journal of Medicine
Obstet Gynecol	Obstetrics and Gynecology
Osteoporos Rev	Osteoporosis Review
Pharm J	Pharmaceutical Journal
Primary Care Resp J	Primary Care Respiratory Journal
Public Health	Public Health
Qual Health Res	Qualitative Health Research
Sex Transm Inf	Sexually Transmitted Infections
Stroke	Stroke
Thorax	Thorax
Tob Control	Tobacco Control
Vaccine	Vaccine

Index